Food Legumes

Food Legumes: Physicochemical and Nutritional Properties

Editor

Ryszard Amarowicz

MDPI • Basel • Beijing • Wuhan • Barcelona • Belgrade • Manchester • Tokyo • Cluj • Tianjin

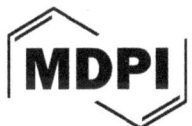

Editor
Ryszard Amarowicz
Polish Academy of Sciences
Poland

Editorial Office
MDPI
St. Alban-Anlage 66
4052 Basel, Switzerland

This is a reprint of articles from the Special Issue published online in the open access journal *Foods* (ISSN 2304-8158) (available at: https://www.mdpi.com/journal/foods/special_issues/Food_Legumes).

For citation purposes, cite each article independently as indicated on the article page online and as indicated below:

LastName, A.A.; LastName, B.B.; LastName, C.C. Article Title. *Journal Name* **Year**, *Volume Number*, Page Range.

ISBN 978-3-0365-1148-1 (Hbk)
ISBN 978-3-0365-1149-8 (PDF)

© 2021 by the authors. Articles in this book are Open Access and distributed under the Creative Commons Attribution (CC BY) license, which allows users to download, copy and build upon published articles, as long as the author and publisher are properly credited, which ensures maximum dissemination and a wider impact of our publications.

The book as a whole is distributed by MDPI under the terms and conditions of the Creative Commons license CC BY-NC-ND.

Contents

About the Editor vii

Preface to "Food Legumes: Physicochemical and Nutritional Properties" ix

Ryszard Amarowicz
Legume Seeds as an Important Component of Human Diet
Reprinted from: *Foods* 2020, 9, 1812, doi: 1

Wojciech Rybiński, Magdalena Karamać, Katarzyna Sulewska, Andreas Börner
and Ryszard Amarowicz
Antioxidant Potential of Grass Pea Seeds from European Countries
Reprinted from: *Foods* 2018, 7, 142, doi: 5

Rayane J. Vital, Priscila Z. Bassinello, Quédma A. Cruz, Rosângela N. Carvalho,
Júlia C. M. de Paiva and Aline O. Colombo
Production, Quality, and Acceptance of Tempeh and White Bean Tempeh Burgers
Reprinted from: *Foods* 2018, 7, 136, doi: 17

Luis Díaz-Batalla, Juan P. Hernández-Uribe, Roberto Gutiérrez-Dorado, Alejandro
Téllez-Jurado, Javier Castro-Rosas, Rogelio Pérez-Cadena and Carlos A. Gómez-Aldapa
Nutritional Characterization of *Prosopis laevigata* Legume Tree (Mesquite) Seed Flour and the
Effect of Extrusion Cooking on its Bioactive Components
Reprinted from: *Foods* 2018, 7, 124, doi: 27

Sabrina Feitosa, Ralf Greiner, Ann-Katrin Meinhardt, Alexandra Müller,
Deusdélia T. Almeida and Clemens Posten
Effect of Traditional Household Processes on Iron, Zinc and Copper Bioaccessibility in Black
Bean (*Phaseolus vulgaris* L.)
Reprinted from: *Foods* 2018, 7, 123, doi: 37

Shayla C. Smithson, Boluwatife D. Fakayode, Siera Henderson, John Nguyen
and Sayo O. Fakayode
Detection, Purity Analysis, and Quality Assurance of Adulterated Peanut (*Arachis hypogaea*) Oils
Reprinted from: *Foods* 2018, 7, 122, doi: 49

Luciane Yuri Yoshiara, Tiago Bervelieri Madeira, Adriano Costa de Camargo,
Fereidoon Shahidi and Elza Iouko Ida
Multistep Optimization of β-Glucosidase Extraction from Germinated Soybeans (*Glycine max* L.
Merril) and Recovery of Isoflavone Aglycones
Reprinted from: *Foods* 2018, 7, 110, doi: 63

About the Editor

Ryszard Amarowicz is Head of the Department of Chemical and Physical Properties of Food and an Editorial Board Member of *Polish Journal of Food and Nutrition Sciences* (Section Editor), *European Journal of Lipid Science, LWT-Food Science and Technology* (Associate Editor), *Food Chemistry, Journal of Food Lipids* (2003–2009), *Food Science and Human Wellness, Foods, Molecules, International Journal of Molecular Sciences, Journal of Food Bioactives*. Prof. Amarowicz is included in the "World's Top 2% Scientists List" by Stanford University, Elsevier, and SciTech Strategies.

Preface to "Food Legumes: Physicochemical and Nutritional Properties"

Legumes are an important source of nutrients (proteins, carbohydrates, water-soluble vitamins, minerals) in human nutrition, and they play important roles in chronic disease prevention. The beneficial effects of legumes are attributed to the presence of legume seed starch, which has a low glycemic index, dietary fiber (soluble and insoluble), several classes of phenolic compounds, and oligosaccharides. Phenolic compounds in legumes possess strong antioxidant and antimicrobial activities. Oligosaccharides, acting as prebiotics, modify intestinal microbiota.

Some of the bioactive compounds present in legumes (e.g., trypsin inhibitors, condensed tannins, lectins, phytates) also exhibit anti-nutritional effects, namely, decreased protein digestibility and availability of mineral compounds. Technological processes (non-thermal and thermal processing, hydrolysis, fractionation) can modify the functional properties (emulsifying activity and stability, foaming properties, water holding capacity) of legumes and legume products, as well as alter the activity of bioactive compounds present in legume seeds.

This new MDPI book publishes important results on phenolic compounds of grass pea and its antioxidant activity; tempeh burgers prepared from white bean and iron, zinc, and copper bioaccessibility in cooked black beans; optimization of the extraction of β-glucosidase from germinated soybeans; the nutritional value of mesquite (legume tree Prosopis laevigata) seed flour and the effect of extrusion cooking on its bioactive components; and the analysis of the purity of highly refined peanut oils that have been adulterated with either vegetable oil, canola oil, or almond oil.

Ryszard Amarowicz
Editor

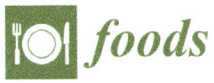

Editorial

Legume Seeds as an Important Component of Human Diet

Ryszard Amarowicz

Institute of Animal Reproduction and Food Research, Polish Academy of Sciences, 10-748 Olsztyn, Poland; r.amarowicz@pan.olsztyn.pl; Tel.:+48-895-234-627; Fax: +48-966-749-677

Received: 3 December 2020; Accepted: 4 December 2020; Published: 7 December 2020

Legumes are an important source of nutrients (proteins, carbohydrates, water soluble vitamins, minerals) for human nutrition. They play important roles in chronic disease prevention. The beneficial effects of legumes are attributed to the presence of legume seed starch with a low glycemic index, dietary fiber (soluble and insoluble), several classes of phenolic compounds, and oligosaccharides [1]. Phenolic compounds of legumes possess strong antioxidant and antimicrobial activities. Oligosaccharides, acting as prebiotics, modify intestinal microbiota [1,2].

Some of the bioactive compounds present in legumes (e.g., trypsin inhibitors, condensed tannins, lectins, phytates) also exhibit anti-nutritional effects—decreased protein digestibility and availability of mineral compounds. Technological processes (non-thermal and thermal processing, hydrolysis, fractionation) can modify the functional properties (emulsifying activity and stability, foaming properties, water holding capacity) of legumes and legume products, as well as modify the activity of bioactive compounds present in legume seeds [1].

Grass pea (*Lathyrus sativus*) exhibits drought tolerance and thrives with minimal external inputs [3]. It is an ideal legume for resource-poor farmers from the Indian subcontinent, Ethiopia and in lesser extent North Africa, Australia, Asia, and Europe [4]. The contents of proteins, starch, lipids, mineral compounds, and energy in grass peas are similar to those of peas and faba bean [5]. Palmitic and linoleic acids are the main fatty acids of grass pea lipids [6]. From a toxicological point of view, the genetic and technological (soaking, cooking, cooking in boiled water at low or high pH) improvement of grass pea is very important for reducing the content of β-N-oxalyl-1-α,β-diamino-propionic acid (β-ODAP) [7]. This non-protein amino acid causes a neurolathyrism, a neurological disease of humans and domestic animals [8].

In the study of Rybiński et al. [9], the total phenolic compound contents of the of 30 varieties of grass pea ranged from 20.3 to 70.3 mg/100 g seeds. The seeds were characterized using Trolox equivalent antioxidant capacity values of 0.158–0.372 mmol Trolox/100 g seeds, and FRAP values of 0.487–1.189 Fe^{2+}/100 g seeds. The total phenolics content of grass pea extract was correlated with the results of the FRAP (ferric-reducing antioxidant power) (r = 0.781) and ABTS (3-ethylbenzothiazoline-6-sulfonic acid) (r = 0.881) assays. The same correlation was observed between the results of both assays (r = 0.842). The authors concluded that grass pea seeds with reduced contents of β-ODAP after technological processing can be a source of phenolic compounds in a vegetarian or vegan diet, and in the general population.

The fermentation of leguminous seeds reduces anti-nutritional compounds, improves protein and starch digestibility, reduces allergenicity, and increases seeds' antioxidant capacity. Therefore, there is a growing interest in promoting the production of fermented leguminous seeds [10]. Tempeh is a traditional Indonesian food, produced by the fermentation of soybeans using *Rhizopus* species, having nutritional qualities and metabolic regulation functions [11].

Vital et al. [12] used white bean (*Phaseolus vilgaris* L.) as a material for tempeh preparation. The results indicated significant differences in the nutritional value of the tempeh produced from white bean and soybean. The produced tempeh samples did not present a risk of microbiological contamination for consumption. The white bean tempeh burgers showed similar appearances and a crispy consistency, but received lower scores for flavor, compared to the soybean burgers. The beany flavor present in white bean tempeh could be minimized by increasing the cooking time of the beans. According to authors, white bean tempeh can be a good alternative for healthy eating, and its manufacture could promote the production of new products made from beans. However, it is still necessary to improve the techniques of production and test new ingredients for the preparation of tempeh burgers to obtain higher acceptability.

Legume seeds are an important source of iron, zinc and copper for human. However Fe, Zn, and Cu absorption is reduced in the presence in seeds of such compounds as phytates and polyphenols, and especially tannins. Technologists recommend seed soaking and discarding the soaking water before cooking, but this leads to mineral loss.

The study of Feitosa et al. [13] aimed to evaluate iron, zinc and copper bioaccessibility in black beans cooked using a regular pan and pressure cooker, with and without the soaking water. The minerals were quantified by inductively coupled plasma mass spectrometry (ICP-MS). In addition, *myo*-inositol phosphates (InsP5, InsP6) were determined by HPLC, and total polyphenols and condensed tannins using colorimetric methods. Mineral bioaccessibility was determined by in vitro digestion and dialysis. All treatments resulted in a statistically significant reduction in total polyphenols (30%) and condensed tannins (20%). Only when discarding the soaking water was a loss of iron (6%) and copper (30%) observed, and InsP6 was slightly decreased (7%) in one treatment. The bioaccessibility values of Fe and Zn were low (about 0.2% iron and 35% zinc). A high bioaccessibility (about 70%) was obtained for cooper. Cooking beans under pressure without discarding the soaking water resulted in the highest bioaccessibility levels among all household procedures. Discarding the soaking water before cooking did not improve the nutritional quality of the beans.

Epicotyls from germinated soybeans (EGS) have great potential as sources of endogenous β-glucosidase. Furthermore, this enzyme may improve the conversion of isoflavones into their corresponding aglycones. This enzyme can also increase the release of aglycones from the cell wall of the plant materials, and epicotyls have been recommended as a potential industrial source of endogenous β-glucosidase [14].

The aim of the work of Yoshiara et al. [15] was to optimize the extraction of β-glucosidase from EGS. Next, the authors examined its application in defatted soybean cotyledon to improve the recovery of aglycones. The optimum extraction of β-glucosidase from EGS occurred at 30 °C and pH 5.0. Furthermore, the maximum recovery of aglycones (98.7%), which occurred at 35 °C and pH 7.0–7.6 during 144 h of germination, increased 8.5 times with respect to the lowest concentration. The higher bioaccessibilty of soybean isoflavone aglycones than that of glucosided was reported by several authors. Therefore, the results obtained may be useful for enhancing the benefits of soybean and soybean products and by-products.

The genus Prosopis is comprised of a group of nitrogen-fixing trees belonging to the Fabaceae family distributed in arid and semiarid regions of Asia, Africa, and America. The pod flour of Prosopis is a versatile ingredient with high potential for the food industry. It is rich in protein, sugars, and fiber, and is gluten-free [16]. One of the important representatives of the genus Prosopis is a legume tree mesquite (*Prosopis laevigata*) that is a widely distributed in Aridoamerica. In the work of Díaz-Batalla et al. [17], the nutritional value of mesquite seed flour and the effect of extrusion cooking on its bioactive components were assessed. The authors found mesquite seed flour to be a rich source of fiber (7.73 g/100 g) and protein (36.51 g/100 g). Valine was the only limiting amino acid of mesquite protein. The total phenolic compound contents in raw and extruded seed flour were 6.68 and 6.46 mg of gallic acid equivalents (GAE)/g, respectively. The high antioxidant potential of mesquite raw and extruded seed flour was confirmed using DPPH assay, and the values were 9.11 and 9.32 mg of ascorbic acid equivalents (AAE)/g, respectively. The extrusion did not generate Maillard reaction product (MRP). The authors found apigenin to be the only flavonoid in mesquite seed flour. This phenolic compound was stable in the extrusion. The authors concluded in their study that mesquite seed flour is a valuable plant food rich in good quality protein and active compounds. The extrusion cooking process of mesquite seed flour is an optional and versatile technology useful in the development of functional foods and the industrialization of this underutilized legume.

Peanut oil is derived from the peanut (*Arachis hypogaea*), a legume that is rich in proteins, vitamins, polyphenols, polyunsaturated fatty acids, and dietary fiber [18,19]. Highly refined peanut oil undergoes several industrial processes, including the extraction of protein allergen, discoloration through bleaching, and deodorization [20].

The study of Smithson et al. [21] reports the analysis of the purity of highly refined peanut oils (HRPO) that were adulterated either with vegetable oil (VO), canola oil (CO), or almond oil (AO) for food quality assurance purposes. It is a fast, simple, accurate, sensitive, and low-cost chemometric approach. The authors used the Fourier transform infrared (FTIR) spectra of the pure oils and adulterated HRPO samples for a partial-least square (PLS) regression analysis. The obtained PLS regression figures-of-merit had very high linearity (R^2 = 0.9942 or higher). The PLS regressions accurately determined the percentage compositions of adulterated HRPOs, with an overall root-mean-square relative percent error of 5.53%, and with the very low limit of detection of 0.02%. The developed PLS regressions continued to predict the compositions of newly prepared adulterated HRPOs over a period of two months, with incredible accuracy without the need for re-calibration. The protocol, due to its sensitivity, accuracy, and robustness, is potentially adoptable.

Funding: This research received no external funding.

Conflicts of Interest: The authors declare no conflict of interest.

References

1. Vaz Patto, M.C.; Amarowicz, R.; Aryee, A.N.A.; Boye, J.I.; Chung, H.-J.; Martín-Cabrejas, M.A.; Domoney, C. Achievements and challenges in improving the nutritional quality of food legumes. *Crit. Rev. Plant. Sci.* **2015**, *34*, 105–143. [CrossRef]
2. Amarowicz, R.; Pegg, R.B. Legumes as a source of natural antioxidants. *Eur. J. Lipid Sci. Technol.* **2008**, *110*, 865–878. [CrossRef]
3. Hillocks, R.J.; Maruthi, M.N. Grass pea (*Lathyrus sativus*): Is there a case for further crop improvement? *Euphytica* **2012**, *186*, 647–654. [CrossRef]
4. Hanbury, C.D.; White, C.L.; Mullan, B.P.; Siddique, K.H.M. A review of the potential of *Lathyrus sativus* L. and *L. cicera* L. grain for use as animal feed. *Anim. Feed Sci. Technol.* **2000**, *87*, 1–27. [CrossRef]
5. Mullan, B.P.; Pluske, J.R.; Trezona, M.; Harris, D.J.; Allen, J.G.; Siddique, K.H.M.; Hanbury, C.D.; van Barneveld, R.J.; Kim, J.C. Chemical composition and standardised ileal digestible amino acid contents of Lathyrus (*Lathyrus cicera*) as an ingredient in pig diets. *Anim. Feed Sci. Technol.* **2009**, *150*, 139–143. [CrossRef]
6. Pastor-Cavada, E.; Jua, R.; Pastor, J.E.; Alai, M.; Vioque, J. Protein isolates from two Mediterranean legumes: *Lathyrus clymenum* and *Lathyrus annuus*. Chemical composition, functional properties and protein characterization. *Food Chem.* **2010**, *122*, 533–538. [CrossRef]
7. Kumar, S.; Bejiga, G.; Ahmed, S.; Nakkoul, H.; Sarker, A. Genetic improvement of grass pea for low neurotoxin (β-ODAP) content. *Food Chem. Toxicol.* **2011**, *49*, 589–600. [CrossRef] [PubMed]
8. Getahun, H.; Lambein, F.; Vanhoorne, M.; Van der Stuyft, P. Pattern and associated factors of the neurolathyrism epidemic in Ethiopia. *Trop. Med. Int. Health* **2002**, *7*, 118–124. [CrossRef] [PubMed]
9. Rybiński, W.; Karamać, M.; Sulewska, K.; Börner, A.; Amarowicz, R. Antioxidant potential of grass pea seeds from European countries. *Foods* **2018**, *7*, 142. [CrossRef] [PubMed]
10. Limón, R.I.; Peñas, E.; Torino, M.I.; Martínez-Villaluenga, C.; Dueñas, M.; Frias, J. Fermentation enhances the content of bioactive compounds in kidney bean extracts. *Food. Chem.* **2015**, *172*, 343–352. [CrossRef] [PubMed]
11. Nakajima, N.; Nozaki, N.; Ishihara, K.; Ishikawa, A.; Tsuji, H. Analysis of isoflavone content in tempeh, a fermented soybean, and preparation of a new isoflavone-enriched tempeh. *J. Biosci. Bioeng.* **2005**, *100*, 685–687. [CrossRef] [PubMed]

12. Vital, R.J.; Bassinello, P.Z.; Cruz, Q.A.; Carvalho, R.N.; De Paiva, J.C.M.; Colombo, A.O. Production, quality, and acceptance of tempeh and white bean tempeh burgers. *Foods* **2018**, *7*, 136. [CrossRef] [PubMed]
13. Feitosa, S.; Ralf Greiner, R.; Ann-Katrin Meinhardt, A.-K.; Alexandra Müller, A.; Deusdélia, T.; Almeida, D.T.; Clemens Posten, C. Effect of traditional household processes on iron, zinc and copper bioaccessibility in black bean (*Phaseolus vulgaris* L.). *Foods* **2018**, *7*, 123. [CrossRef] [PubMed]
14. Yoshiara, L.Y.; Madeira, T.B.; Ribeiro, M.L.L.; Mandarino, J.M.G.; Carrão-Panizzi, M.C.; Ida, E.I. β-Glucosidase activity of soybean (*Glycine max*) embryonic axis germinated in the presence or absence of light. *J. Food Biochem.* **2011**, *36*, 699–705. [CrossRef]
15. Yoshiara, L.Y.; Madeira, T.B.; De Camargo, A.C.; Shahidi, F.; Ida, E.I. Multistep optimization of β-glucosidase extraction from germinated soybeans (*Glycine max* L. Merril) and recovery of isoflavone aglycones. *Foods* **2018**, *7*, 110. [CrossRef]
16. Felker, P.; Takeoka, G.; Dao, L. Pod mesocarp flour of north and south american species of leguminous tree Prosopis (Mesquite): Composition and food applications. *Food Rev. Int.* **2013**, *29*, 49–66. [CrossRef]
17. Díaz-Batalla, L.; Hernández-Uribe, J.P.; Gutiérrez-Dorado, R.; Téllez-Jurado, A.; Castro-Rosas, J.; Pérez-Cadena, R.; Gómez-Aldapa, C.A. Nutritional characterization of prosopis laevigata legume tree (Mesquite) seed flour and the effect of extrusion cooking on its bioactive components. *Foods* **2018**, *7*, 124. [CrossRef]
18. Carrín, M.E.; Carelli, A.A. Peanut oil: Compositional data. *Eur. J. Lipid Sci. Technol.* **2010**, *112*, 697–707. [CrossRef]
19. Lusas, E.W. Food uses of peanut protein. *J. Am. Oil Chem. Soc.* **1979**, *56*, 425–430. [CrossRef] [PubMed]
20. List, G.R. Processing and Food Uses of Peanut Oil and Protein. In *Peanut: Genetics, Processing, and Utilization*; Academic Press and AOCS Press: Washington, IL, USA, 2016; pp. 405–428.
21. Smithson, S.C.; Boluwatife, D.; Fakayode, B.D.; Henderson, S.; John Nguyen, J.; Fakayode, S.O. Detection, purity analysis, and quality assurance of adulterated peanut (*Arachis hypogaea*) oils. *Foods* **2018**, *7*, 122. [CrossRef] [PubMed]

Publisher's Note: MDPI stays neutral with regard to jurisdictional claims in published maps and institutional affiliations.

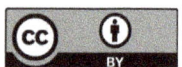

© 2020 by the author. Licensee MDPI, Basel, Switzerland. This article is an open access article distributed under the terms and conditions of the Creative Commons Attribution (CC BY) license (http://creativecommons.org/licenses/by/4.0/).

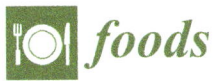

Article

Antioxidant Potential of Grass Pea Seeds from European Countries

Wojciech Rybiński [1], Magdalena Karamać [2], Katarzyna Sulewska [2], Andreas Börner [3] and Ryszard Amarowicz [2,*]

1. Institute of Plant Genetics, Polish Academy of Sciences, Strzeszyńska 34, 60-479 Poznań, Poland; wryb@igr.poznan.pl
2. Institute of Animal Reproduction and Food Research, Polish Academy of Sciences, 10-748 Olsztyn, Poland; m.karamac@pan.olsztyn.pl (M.K.), k.sulewska@pan.olsztyn.pl (K.S.)
3. Leibniz Institute of Plant Genetics and Crop Plant Research, D-06466 Gatersleben, Germany; boerner@ipk-gatersleben.de
* Correspondence: r.amarowicz@pan.olsztyn.pl; Tel.: +48-895-2346-27

Received: 6 July 2018; Accepted: 27 August 2018; Published: 1 September 2018

Abstract: Phenolic compounds were extracted from seeds of 30 varieties of grass pea (*Lathyrus sativus*) into 80% (v/v) methanol. The total phenolics compounds content of the extracts and their antioxidant activity were determined using Folin-Ciocalteu's phenol reagent and 2,2′-azinobis-(3-ethylbenzothiazoline-6-sulfonic acid) (ABTS) and ferric-reducing antioxidant power (FRAP) methods, respectively. Total phenolic contents ranged from 1.88 to 7.12 mg/g extract and 20.3 to 70.3 mg/100 g seeds. The extracts and seeds were characterized using Trolox equivalent antioxidant capacity values of 0.015–0.037 mmol Trolox/g extract and 0.158–0.372 mmol Trolox/100 g seeds, and FRAP values of 0.045–0.120 mmol Fe^{2+}/g extract and 0.487–1.189 Fe^{2+}/100 g seeds. The total phenolics content of grass pea extract was correlated with the results of the ABTS ($r = 0.881$) and FRAP ($r = 0.781$) assays. The same correlation was observed between the results of both assays ($r = 0.842$). Two derivatives of *p*-coumaric acid were the dominant phenolic compounds of the Derek cultivar of grass pea.

Keywords: grass pea; *Lathyrus sativus*; phenolic compounds; antioxidant activity

1. Introduction

Grass pea (*Lathyrus sativus*) is an ideal legume for resource-poor farmers, characterized by drought tolerance and thriving with minimal external inputs [1]. It is cultivated in the Indian subcontinent, Ethiopia, and to a lesser extent in North Africa, Australia, Asia, and Europe [2]. Currently, grass peas, similar to other legumes such as chickpea, lentil, and vetch are beginning to be cultivated in the Old World [3]. Grass pea seeds have a high nutritional value [4]. The protein, starch, lipids, mineral, and energy content in grass peas is similar to those of peas and faba beans [5]. For example, according to literature data, the protein content in grass pea, pea, and faba bean seeds is 26.5, 20.6, and 19–30 g/100 g, respectively [5–7]. The fatty acid profile of grass pea lipids is valuable. A high percentage of stearic acid was determined in grass pea lipids by Mehmet [8]. In epidemiologic and clinical studies, stearic acid was found to be associated with lowered low-density lipoprotein (LDL) cholesterol in comparison with other saturated fatty acids [9].

Unfortunately, grass pea seeds contain a neurotoxin, β-*N*-oxalyl-1-α,β-diamino-propionic acid (β-ODAP). This non-protein amino acid causes neurolathyrism, a neurological disease in humans and domestic animals [10]. The β-ODAP content of traditional grass pea cultivars is 0.5–2.5%. Genetic improvement of grass pea has reduced this content to <0.10% [11]. Soaking and boiling considerably reduces the content of β-ODAP in grass pea seeds [12,13]. Grass pea seeds can be used as a high-value protein source after protein extraction and the removal of antinutritional components [14].

Suitable functional properties (water absorption capacity, oil absorption capacity, foaming capacity, and foaming stability) of grass pea proteins were reported by Aletor et al. [15].

Legumes are a potentially valuable crop with high antioxidant potential [16]. The antioxidant and antiradical activities of leguminous seed extracts have been investigated using a variety of methods including liposomes, enhanced chemiluminescence, a β-carotene-linoleate model system, 2,2′-diphenyl-1-picrylhydrazyl (DPPH) and 2,2′-azinobis-(3-ethylbenzothiazoline-6-sulfonic acid) ABTS assays, the reducing power assay, LDL cholesterol oxidation, ferric-reducing antioxidant power (FRAP) assay, Fe^{2+}-chelating capacity assay, and the hydrophilic oxygen radical absorbance capacity ($ORAC_{FL}$) assay [17].

The reported content of total phenolics of grass pea flour was 0.22 and 0.27 g/100 g [18]. The phenolic content of grass pea extracts was correlated with their antioxidant properties determined using DPPH, FRAP, and β-carotene bleaching methods [19]. Menga et al. [20] reported linear correlations between the content of total phenolics, total flavonoids, and condensed tannins and results of the ABTS assay for grass pea extracts ($p < 0.001$). Total phenolic and condensed tannin levels were not correlated with seed yield and seed protein content in grass pea [21]. Grass peas extract inhibited α-amylase and α-glucosidase in an in vitro bioassay [19]. Results obtained by Stanisavljević et al. [22] strongly suggest that simple cooking treatment and in vitro digestion of grass pea seed flour applied prior to extraction with methanol could improve the antioxidative activity of the obtained extracts.

The present study aimed to determine the total phenolic content of grass pea extracts and seeds as well their antioxidant activity and potential. To the best of our knowledge, this is the first publication to consider such a broad biological material from several countries.

2. Materials and Methods

2.1. Plant Material

Plant material consisted of a collection of 30 grass pea varieties obtained in a field experiment conducted in Cerekwica (51°55′ N, 17°21′ E) derived from Italian, Spanish, French, German, and Polish lines. Descriptors for *Lathyrus sativus* were used (IPGRI 2000) for the evaluation and characterization of the phenotypic features of the new lines. The growth habit of each line was recorded at 50% flowering and scored as prostrate, spreading, semi-erect or erect. Flower colors were scored as blue, pink, red, white, or various combination of these colours. Pod shapes were scored as oblong, medium, oblong elliptical, curved, broad, broad-linear/elliptical, or a combination of these shapes. Seed coat color and shape were recorded on 100 randomly selected seeds immediately after threshing. Seed shape was generally classified as angled or wedge-shaped. After harvest, 10 randomly selected plants from each accession were chosen for estimation of quantitative traits (yield structure parameters). The weight of 100 seeds was calculated from weighing and counting at least 200 seeds. Until extraction, the seeds were stored in a refrigerator closed in vacuum bags. The characteristics of those seeds are reported in Table 1.

Table 1. Characteristic of grass seeds investigated in this study.

No.	Accession Code	Country of Origin	Seeds Coat Color	Weight of 100 Seeds (g)
1	LAT 4051/99	Italy	Cream to bright green	37.8
2	LAT 4052/99	Italy	Cream to bright green	42.6
3	LAT 4053/99	Italy	Cream to bright green	28.2
4	LAT 4054/99	Italy	Cream, mottled with brown edge	25.7
5	LAT 4055/99	Italy	Cream, slightly mottled and flattened	46.5
6	LAT 4056/99	Italy	Green	29.0
7	LAT 4061/99	Italy	Greyed-white with brown edge	32.1
8	LAT 4063/01	Italy	Cream-white	29.1
9	LAT 4064/01	Italy	Brick-red, dark mottled	30.0

Table 1. Cont.

No.	Accession Code	Country of Origin	Seeds Coat Color	Weight of 100 Seeds (g)
10	LAT 4065/01	Italy	Greyed-white with brown edge	24.9
11	LAT 4068/01	Italy	Brick-red, dark mottled	29.4
12	LAT 4069/01	Italy	Cream slightly flattened	30.4
13	LAT 4070/01	Italy	Brick-red, dark mottled	24.7
14	LAT 4071/01	Italy	Cream	20.1
15	LAT 4074/01	Italy	Greyed-white with brown edge	30.0
16	LAT 4075/00	Italy	Cream with brown edge	31.3
17	LAT 4078/00	Italy	Cream to bright green with brown edge	48.0
18	LAT 4079/01	Italy	Cream with brown edge	40.9
19	LAT 4081/00	Italy	Cream	18.2
20	LAT 4082/00	Italy	Cream with brown edge	21.4
21	LAT 456/75	Spain	Cream with dark edge	28.5
22	LAT 1706/92	Spain	Cream with short black edge	27.7
23	LAT 4006/84	Spain	Cream with brown edge	23.5
24	LAT 4007/84	Spain	Cream	25.3
25	LAT 4085/73	Spain	Cream	26.1
26	LAT 444/73	Germany	Cream, brown edge, slightly mottled	16,7
27	LAT 478	Germany	Gray, dark brown edge, slightly mottled	19.5
28	LAT 447	France	Cream, slightly brick-red	16.4
29	LAT 448	France	Cream	17.9
30	Cultivar Derek	Poland	Bridge-cream	11.8

LAT means "*Lathyrus*". Seed size (100 seeds): below 15 g: small; 15–25 g: medium, and above 25 g: large.

2.2. Chemicals

Sodium persulfate, ferrous chloride, Folin-Ciocalteau's phenol reagent, 2,2′-azinobis-(3-ethylbenzothiazoline-6-sulfonic acid) (ABTS), 2,4,6-tri(2-pyridyl)-*s*-triazine (TPTZ), 6-hydroxy-2,5,7,8-tetramethyl-chroman-2-carboxylic acid (Trolox), and (+)-catechin were purchased from Sigma (Poznań, Poland). Acetonitrile high-performance liquid chromatography (HPLC) grade and methanol were obtained from P.O.Ch. Company (Gliwice, Poland).

2.3. Extraction

Phenolic compounds were extracted from ground seeds using 80% (v/v) methanol at a solids to solvent ratio of 1:10 (w/v) for 15 min at 50 °C [23]. The extraction was repeated twice, the supernatants were filtered and combined, and methanol was evaporated under vacuum in a R-200 rotary evaporator (Büchi Labortechnik AG, Flawil, Switzerland). The remaining aqueous solution was lyophilized.

2.4. Total Phenolic Compounds Content

The method described by Naczk and Shahidi [24] was used to determine the total phenolic compounds content of the extracts. Briefly, a 0.5-mL aliquot of seed extract dissolved in methanol was pipetted into a test tube containing 8 mL distilled water. After mixing the contents, 0.5 mL Folin-Ciocalteu's phenol reagent and 1 mL saturated sodium carbonate solution were added. The contents were vortexed for 15 s and then left to stand at room temperature for 30 min. Absorbance measurements were recorded at 725 nm using a Beckman DU 7500 Spectrophotometer (Beckman Poland, Warsaw, Poland). Estimation of the phenolic compounds was carried out in triplicate. The results are expressed as (+)-catechin equivalents per g of the extract or 100 g seeds.

2.5. Condensed Tannins

Condensed tannins were determined using a vanillin/HCL colorimetric method [25]. The results obtained are reported as absorbance units at 500 nm per 1 mg extract.

2.6. ABTS Assay

The Trolox equivalent antioxidant capacity (TEAC) was determined using a method described by Re et al. [26]. Here, ABTS$^+$ solution was prepared by mixing an ABTS stock solution in water with 2.45 mM sodium persulphate. This mixture was allowed to stand with shaking for 12–16 h at room temperature in the dark until reaching a stable oxidative state. For analysis, the ABTS$^+$ stock solution was diluted with methanol to an absorbance of 0.720 at 734 nm. For the spectrophotometric assay, 2 mL ABTS$^+$ reagent and 20 µL plant extract were mixed and the absorbance was read at 734 nm at 37 °C for 10 min. A calibration curve was plotted using Trolox standard solution. The results are expressed as mmol Trolox equivalent per g extract or 100 g seeds.

2.7. Ferric-Reducing Antioxidant Power (FRAP) Assay

The ferric-reducing antioxidant power (FRAP) assay was performed as previously described by Benzie and Strain [27]. The sample solution was first diluted with deionized water to fit within the linearity range. The working FRAP reagent was prepared by mixing 10 volumes of 300 mM acetate buffer, pH 3.6, with 1 volume of 10 mM TPTZ in 40 mM HCL, and with 1 volume of 20 mM FeCl$_3$ × 6H$_2$O. A volume of 2.25 mL of a working FRAP reagent was warmed to 37 °C. Then, 75 µL of the sample and 225 µL of deionized water were added to the FRAP reagent and the absorbance was measured at 593 nm against a reagent blank after 30 min incubation. The FRAP values were calculated and are expressed as mmol of Fe^{2+} equivalent per g extract or 100 g of seeds.

2.8. HPLC Analysis

Methanolic extract (20 mg) of Derek cultivar was dissolved in 2 mL of 80% methanol and filtered through a 0.45 µm cellulose acetate filter (Millipore, Warsaw, Poland). Phenolic compounds were analysed using a Shimadzu HPLC system (Shimadzu Corp., Kyoto, Japan) consisting of two LC-10AD pumps, a SCTL 10A system controller, and a SPD-M 10A photodiode array detector. The chromatography was performed using a pre-packed Luna C18 column (4 × 250 mm, 5 µm; Phenomenex, Torrance, CA, USA). Elution proceeded for 50 min in a gradient system of 5–40% acetonitrile in water adjusted to pH 2.5 with trifluoroacetic acid (TFA) [28]; the detector was set at 320, the injection volume was 20 µL, and the flow rate was 1 mL/min.

2.9. Statistical Analysis

The results obtained in this study are reported as the mean values of three estimates ± standard deviation. Pearson correlation was used to determine the relationship between total phenolics content, TEAC, and FRAP. Principal component analysis (PCA) and hierarchical cluster analysis (HCA) with Ward's method using Euclidean distances were also used. Statistical and chemometric data analyses were performed using Statistica (Windows software package 8.0, Dell Inc., Tulsa, OK, USA).

3. Results and Discussion

3.1. Content of Total Phenolics Compounds

The total phenolics contents of the extracts were determined using a Folin-Ciocalteu's phenol reagent. The results are expressed as (+)-catechin equivalents per g of the extract or 100 g seeds (Table 2). The total phenolic content ranged from 1.88 (LAT 4065/01) to 7.12 mg/g extract (LAT 4054/99) and from 20.3 (LAT 4065/01) to 70.3 mg/100 g seeds (LAT 4065/01). These concentrations are low and can be compared to those obtained previously for white bean [28] and pea [16]. Very similar total phenolic contents (20.6 and 21.3 mg/100g) were reported by Fratianni et al. [29] in two Italian varieties of grass pea, and by Wang et al. [21].in nine varieties of Canadian grass pea (16.2–37.5 mg/100 g). Higher total phenolic compounds contents in grass pea were reported by Wiszniewska and Piwowarczyk [30] and Carbonaro et al. [18].

Table 2. Characteristics of the grass pea seeds and their extracts: content of total phenolics and antioxidant activity.

No.	Total Phenolics [1]		ABTS [2] Assay		FRAP [3] Assay	
	mg/g Extract	mg/100 g Seeds	mmol TE/g Extract	mmol TE/100 g Seeds	mmol Fe^{2+}/g Extract	mmol Fe^{2+}/100 g Seeds
1	3.49 ± 0.07	40.6 ± 0.8	0.015 ± 0.000	0.170 ± 0.001	0.074 ± 0.001	0.859 ± 0.009
2	3.85 ± 0.04	41.6 ± 0.4	0.020 ± 0.000	0.214 ± 0.001	0.080 ± 0.002	0.861 ± 0.021
3	2.63 ± 0.03	30.5 ± 0.4	0.016 ± 0.000	0.186 ± 0.003	0.061 ± 0.001	0.713 ± 0.017
4	7.12 ± 0.10	73.0 ± 1.1	0.037 ± 0.001	0.372 ± 0.014	0.120 ± 0.001	1.028 ± 0.012
5	3.12 ± 0.04	36.1 ± 0.4	0.022 ± 0.000	0.253 ± 0.001	0.073 ± 0.002	0.851 ± 0.021
6	2.40 ± 0.03	27.2 ± 0.4	0.016 ± 0.000	0.176 ± 0.001	0.058 ± 0.001	0.654 ± 0.010
7	3.66 ± 0.04	48.2 ± 0.5	0.018 ± 0.000	0.241 ± 0.003	0.059 ± 0.001	0.780 ± 0.015
8	3.68 ± 0.02	41.6 ± 0.2	0.019 ± 0.000	0.210 ± 0.004	0.059 ± 0.001	0.662 ± 0.004
9	6.35 ± 0.10	65.5 ± 1.0	0.031 ± 0.001	0.319 ± 0.0013	0.115 ± 0.001	1.189 ± 0.008
10	1.88 ± 0.07	20.3 ± 0.8	0.015 ± 0.000	0.232 ± 0.002	0.045 ± 0.003	0.487 ± 0.002
11	3.97 ± 0.17	41.6 ± 1.8	0.022 ± 0.000	0.158 ± 0.002	0.084 ± 0.002	0.889 ± 002
12	1.99 ± 0.05	22.1 ± 0.6	0.017 ± 0.000	0.191 ± 0.004	0.101 ± 0.002	0.557 ± 0.008
13	5.68 ± 0.10	61.8 ± 1.1	0.033 ± 0.001	0.229 ± 0.002	0.069 ± 0.002	1.105 ± 0.002
14	4.11 ± 0.09	42.4 ± 0.9	0.026 ± 0.001	0.232 ± 0.002	0.069 ± 0.001	0.707 ± 0.024
15	4.45 ± 0.07	45.0 ± 0.7	0.031 ± 0.001	0.309 ± 0.002	0.083 ± 0.002	0.835 ± 0.018
16	3.94 ± 0.03	38.6 ± 0.3	0.023 ± 0.000	0.225 ± 0.002	0.074 ± 0.001	0.724 ± 0.006
17	3.24 ± 0.03	37.4 ± 0.4	0.020 ± 0.000	0.229 ± 0.001	0.063 ± 0.002	0.728 ± 0.021
18	4.18 ± 0.07	47.2 ± 0.7	0.020 ± 0.000	0.227 ± 0.001	0.062 ± 0.002	0.698 ± 0.021
19	5.37 ± 0.07	56.8 ± 0.7	0.025 ± 0.001	0.263 ± 0.004	0.073 ± 0.001	0.769 ± 0.006
20	4.84 ± 0.03	49.5 ± 0.7	0.028 ± 0.001	0.284 ± 0.006	0.073 ± 0.001	0.740 ± 0.012
21	3.27 ± 0.04	35.7 ± 0.4	0.016 ± 0.000	0.179 ± 0.001	0.060 ± 0.003	0.524 ± 0.030
22	4.24 ± 0.07	46.9 ± 0.8	0.024 ± 0.001	0.269 ± 0.001	0.062 ± 0.001	0.678 ± 0.09
23	4.55 ± 0.07	48.0 ± 0.3	0.022 ± 0.000	0.230 ± 0.004	0.060 ± 0.001	0.655 ± 0.010
24	3.50 ± 0.04	36.9 ± 0.3	0.019 ± 0.000	0.196 ± 0.003	0.053 ± 0.002	0.557 ± 0.018
25	2.45 ± 0.03	37.4 ± 0.5	0.016 ± 0.000	0.180 ± 0.003	0.059 ± 0.002	0.687 ± 0.030
26	4.40 ± 0.06	41.4 ± 0.7	0.021 ± 0.000	0.212 ± 0.004	0.062 ± 0.002	0.622 ± 0.024
27	4.82 ± 0.10	59.1 ± 0.7	0.027 ± 0.001	0.293 ± 0.006	0.062 ± 0.003	0.683 ± 0.028
28	2.49 ± 0.07	49.7 ± 0.3	0.020 ± 0.000	0.205 ± 0.007	0.070 ± 0.003	0.723 ± 0.031
29	4.77 ± 0.11	32.5 ± 0.4	0.025 ± 0.001	0.244 ± 0.004	0.066 ± 0.001	0.659 ± 0.010
30	2.26 ± 0.02	41.3 ± 0.7	0.019 ± 0.000	0.180 ± 0.001	0.065 ± 0.001	0.638 ± 0.007

[1] As (+)-catechin equivalents; [2] 2,2′-azinobis-(3-ethylbenzothiazoline-6-sulfonic acid); [3] Ferric-Reducing Antioxidant Power.

3.2. Content of Condensed Tannins

The extracts obtained from samples 5, 10, 12, 16, 17, 21, 22, 23, and 28 contained small amounts of condensed tannins. The results expressed as absorbance at 500 nm per mg extract ranged from 0.001 to 0.004. The contents of condensed tannins reported previously for extracts of lentil, abzuki bean, faba bean, broad bean, and red bean were much higher [16].

3.3. Antioxidant Activity

The results of the ABTS and FRAP assays are presented in Table 2. The extracts and seeds were characterized by the Trolox equivalent antioxidant capacity (TEAC) values, ranging from 0.015 (LAT 4051/99 and LAT 4065/01) to 0.037 mmol Trolox/g extract (LAT 4054/99) and from 0.158 (LAT 4068/01) to 0.372 mmol Trolox/100 g seeds (LAT 4054/99). Ferric-reducing antioxidant power (FRAP) values varied from 0.045 (LAT 4065/01) to 0.120 mmol Fe^{2+}/g extract (LAT 4054/99) and from 0.487 (LAT 4068/01) to 1.189 Fe^{2+}/100 g seeds (LAT 4054/99). The results were compared to those reported previously for white bean [16,23]. Some papers reported the antioxidant capacity of grass pea seeds or their extracts determined using DPPH, ABTS, and FRAP assays, β-carotene bleaching, and H_2O_2 scavenge [22,31–33]. In general, the results were lower relative to the results reported for other leguminous seeds. For example, extracts of cow pea were characterised by TEAC and TRAP values of 0.285–0.665 TE/g extract and 0.487–1.560 mmol Fe^{2+}/g extract [34].

3.4. HPLC Analysis

The phenolic compounds contained in grass pea of the Derek cultivar were separated by HPLC, and the resulting chromatogram showed the presence of two major peaks (1 and 2) with retention times of 20.5 and 26.4 min, respectively (Figure 1). The UV-diode array detector (UV-DAD) spectra of compound 1 were characterized by maxima at 309 nm and were very similar to the spectrum of *p*-coumaric acid (Figure 2). The contents of compounds 1 and 2 in the extract and seeds of Derek cultivar are reported in Table 3. The presence of *p*-coumaric acid and its derivatives have been reported for lentil, broad bean, adzuki bean, and faba bean [35–38]. The high content of *p*-coumaric acid in grass pea was reported by Carbonaro et al. [18].

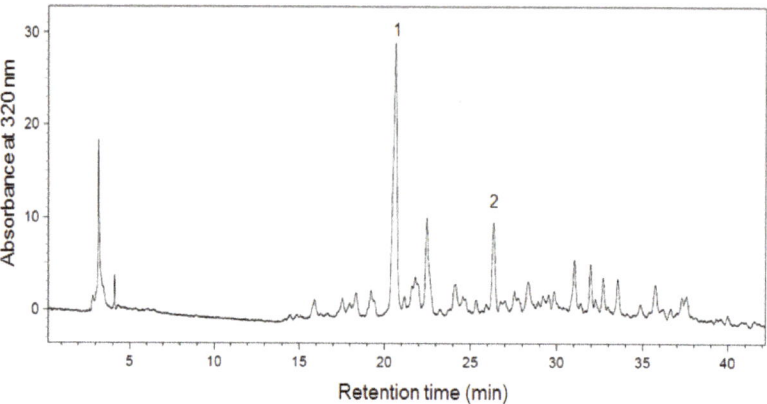

Figure 1. High performance liquid chromatography (HPLC) chromatogram of *Lathyrus sativus* Derek cultivar extract.

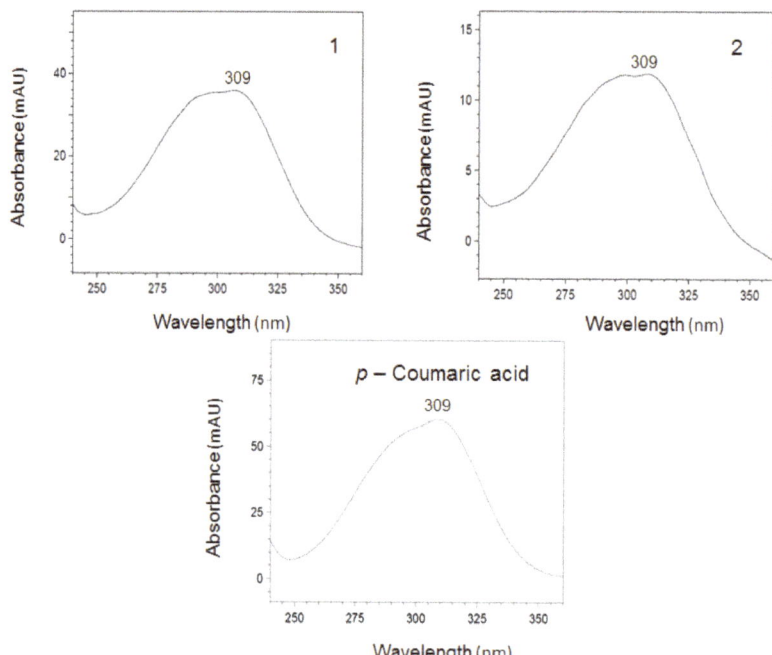

Figure 2. UV-diode array detector (UV-DAD) spectra of compound 1 and 2 separated using HPLC method and standard of *p*-coumaric acid.

Table 3. Content of two main phenolic compounds in Derek cultivar of grass pea.

Phenolic Compound	Content [1]	
	mg/g Extract	mg/g 100 g Seeds
1	1.15 ± 0.05	20.7 ± 2.7
2	0.48 ± 0.03	8.64 ± 0.54

[1] *p*-coumaric acid equivalents.

3.5. Statistical Analysis

In this work, for the first time, a correlation was calculated between the content of phenolic compounds in the grass pea extracts and their antioxidant activity. The correlation coefficients between the total phenolics content and the results of the ABTS and FRAP assays were 0.881 and 0.781, respectively. This correlation was also observed in the results of both assays (r = 0.842) (Figure 3). A similar relationship between the content of total phenolics in leguminous extracts and their antioxidant activities was previously reported by Amarowicz et al. [39] and Orac et al. [28,40].

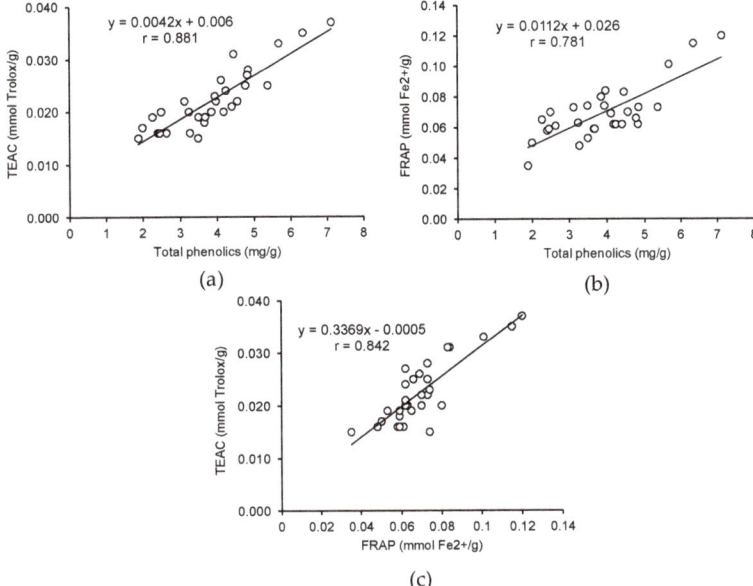

Figure 3. Correlation between (**a**) the total phenolics content and the results of 2,2′-azinobis-(3-ethylb enzothiazoline-6-sulfonic acid) (ABTS) assay, (**b**) total phenolics content and the results of the ferric-reducing antioxidant power (FRAP) assay, and (**c**) results of the two antioxidant assays.

In the principal component analysis (PCA) (Figure 4), the two first components accounted for 90.3% of the total variability between the grass pea varieties. The considerable variability in terms of the analyzed traits expressed jointly with the greatest Mahalanobis distance was recorded for Italian samples 3, 4, 9, 10, and 13 (LAT 4053/99, LAT 4054/99, LAT 4064/01, LAT 4065/01, and LAT 4070/01, respectively). According to Figure 2, discrimination of the sample geographical origin by PCA was rather difficult.

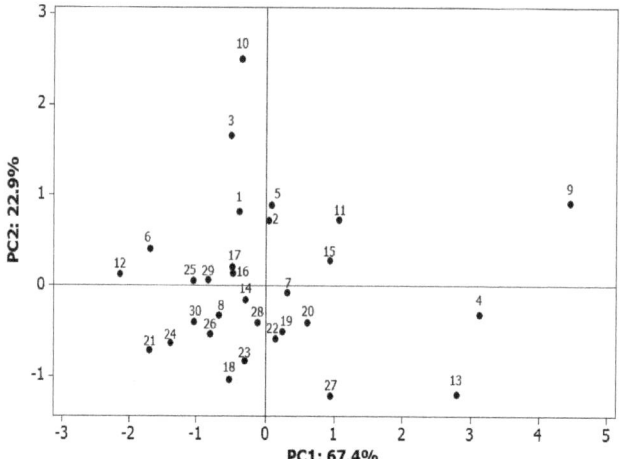

Figure 4. Results of the principal component analysis (PCA).

The hierarchical cluster analysis (Figure 5) shows several pairs of grass pea accessions (e.g., LAT 4053/99 and LAT 448; LAT 4061/01 and LAT 4006/84). Several of these pairs are, in turn, similar to each other (e.g., pair LAT 4061/01 and LAT 4006/84 and pair LAT 4063/10 and LAT 1706/92), whereas LAT 4054/99 is entirely different from all the others. The presence of similar pairs of grass peas accessions from different countries confirms the limitation of the hierarchical cluster analysis for the discrimination of the sample geographical origin.

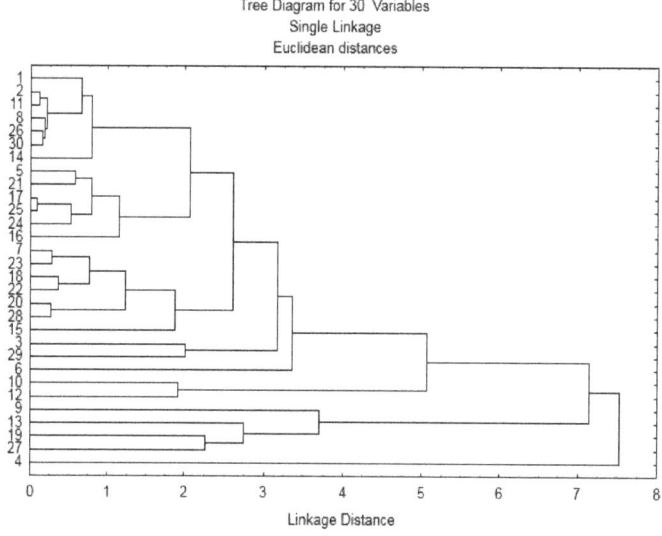

Figure 5. The hierarchical cluster analysis.

4. Conclusions

Grass pea seeds with reduced content of β-ODAP after technological processing can be a source of phenolic compounds in a vegetarian or vegan diet, and in the general population. The contents of total phenolics in grass pea extract are correlated, as demonstrated by the results of the ABTS and FRAP assays. The correlation was also observed between results of both assays. Two derivatives of *p*-coumaric acid were the dominant phenolic compounds of the Derek cultivar of grass pea. In future studies, the bioavailability of grass pea phenolic compounds will be investigated in vitro.

Author Contributions: W.R. Conceptualization, produced and contributed plant material, wrote the study; M.K. Performed the statistical analysis and wrote the study; K.S. Formal analysis; A.B. Produced and contributed plant material; R.A. Conceptualization and wrote the study.

Funding: This research received no external funding.

Acknowledgments: The technical assistance of Kamila Penkacik is acknowledged.

Conflicts of Interest: The authors declare no conflict of interest.

References

1. Hillocks, R.J.; Maruthi, M.N. Grass pea (*Lathyrus sativus*): Is there a case for further crop improvement? *Euphytica* **2012**, *186*, 647–654. [CrossRef]
2. Hanbury, C.D.; White, C.L.; Mullan, B.P.; Siddique, K.H.M. A review of the potential of *Lathyrus sativus* L. and *L. cicera* L. grain for use as animal feed. *Anim. Feed Sci. Technol.* **2000**, *87*, 1–27. [CrossRef]
3. Mikić, A.; Mihailović, V.; Ćupina, B.; Ethurić, B.; Krstić, D.; Vasić, M.; Vasiljević, S.; Karagi, D.; Dorthević, V. Towards the re-introduction of grass pea (*Lathyrus sativus*) in the West Balkan countries: The case of Serbia and Srpska (Bosnia and Herzegovina). *Food Chem. Toxicol.* **2011**, *49*, 650–654.
4. Ennenking, D. The nutritive value of grass pea (*Lathyrus sativus*) and allied species, their toxicity to animals and the role of malnutrition in neurolathyrism. *Food Chem. Toxicol.* **2011**, *49*, 694–709. [CrossRef] [PubMed]
5. Mullan, B.P.; Pluske, J.R.; Trezona, M.; Harris, D.J.; Allen, J.G.; Siddique, K.H.M.; Hanbury, C.D.; van Barneveld, R.J.; Kim, J.C. Chemical composition and standardised ileal digestible amino acid contents of Lathyrus (*Lathyrus cicera*) as an ingredient in pig diets. *Anim. Feed Sci. Technol.* **2009**, *150*, 139–143. [CrossRef]
6. Wozniak, A.; Soroka, M.; Stepniowska, A. Chemical composition of pea (*Pisum sativum* L.) seeds depending on tillage systems. *J. Elementol.* **2014**, *14*, 1143–1152. [CrossRef]
7. Kumar, A.; Nidhi, P.; Sinha, S.K. Nutritional and antinutritional attributes of faba bean (*Vicia faba* L.) germ plasms growing in Bihar, India. *Physiol. Mol. Biol. Plants* **2015**, *21*, 159–162. [CrossRef] [PubMed]
8. Mehmet, A. Fatty acid characteristics of grass pea (*Lathyrus sativus*) in an East Mediterranean environment. *Cogent Chem.* **2017**, *3*. [CrossRef]
9. Hunter, J.E.; Zhang, J.; Kris-Etherton, P.M. Cardiovascular disease risk of dietary stearic acid compared with trans, other saturated, and unsaturated fatty acids: A systematic review. *Am. J. Clin. Nutr.* **2009**, *91*, 46–63. [CrossRef] [PubMed]
10. Getahun, H.; Lambein, F.; Vanhoorne, M.; Van der Stuyft, P. Pattern and associated factors of the neurolathyrism epidemic in Ethiopia. *Trop. Med. Int. Health* **2002**, *7*, 118–124. [CrossRef] [PubMed]
11. Kumar, S.; Bejiga, G.; Ahmed, S.; Nakkoul, H.; Sarker, A. Genetic improvement of grass pea for low neurotoxin (β-ODAP) content. *Food Chem. Toxicol.* **2011**, *49*, 589–600. [CrossRef] [PubMed]
12. Khandare, A.L.; Kumar, R.H.; Meshram, I.I.; Arlappa, N.; Laxmaiah, A.; Venkaiah, K.; Rao, P.A.; Validandi, V.; Toteja, G.S. Current scenario of consumption of *Lathyrus sativus* and lathyrism in three districts of Chhattisgarh State, India. *Toxicon* **2018**, *150*, 228–234. [CrossRef] [PubMed]
13. Srivastava, S.; Khokhar, S. Effect of processing on the reduction of β-ODAP (β-*N*-Oxalyl-L-2,3-diaminopropionic acid) and anti-nutrients of khesari dhal, *Lathyrus sativus*. *J. Sci. Food Agric.* **1996**, *71*, 50–58. [CrossRef]
14. Pastor-Cavada, E.; Jua, R.; Pastor, J.E.; Alai, M.; Vioque, J. Protein isolates from two Mediterranean legumes: *Lathyrus clymenum* and *Lathyrus annuus*. Chemical composition, functional properties and protein characterization. *Food Chem.* **2010**, *122*, 533–538. [CrossRef]
15. Aletor, O.; Onyemem, C.E.; Aletor, V.A. Nutrient constituents, functional attributes and in vitro protein digestibility of the seeds of the *Lathyrus* plant. *WIT Trans. Ecol. Environ.* **2011**, *152*, 145–155. [CrossRef]
16. Amarowicz, R.; Pegg, R.B. Legumes as a source of natural antioxidants. *Eur. J. Lipid Sci. Technol.* **2008**, *110*, 865–878. [CrossRef]

17. Vaz Patto, M.C.; Amarowicz, R.; Aryee, A.N.A.; Boye, J.I.; Chung, H.-J.; Martín-Cabrejas, M.A.; Domoney, C. Achievements and challenges in improving the nutritional quality of food legumes. *Crit. Rev. Plant. Sci.* **2015**, *34*, 105–143. [CrossRef]
18. Carbonaro, M.; Nardini, M.; Maselli, P.; Nucara, A. Chemico-physical and nutritional properties of traditional legumes (lentil, *Lens culinaris* L., and grass pea, *Lathyrus sativus* L.) from organic agriculture: An explorative study. *Org. Agric.* **2015**, *5*, 179–292. [CrossRef]
19. Talukdar, D. Antioxidant potential and type II diabetes related enzyme inhibition properties of raw and processed legumes in Indian Himalayas. *J. Appl. Pharm. Sci.* **2013**, *3*, 13–19. [CrossRef]
20. Menga, V.; Codianni, P.; Fares, C. Agronomic management under organic farming may affect the bioactive compounds of lentil (*Lens culinaris* L.) and grass pea (*Lathyrus communis* L.)? *Sustainability* **2014**, *6*, 1059–1075. [CrossRef]
21. Wang, X.; Warkentin, T.D.; Briggs, C.J.; Granese, T.; Albanese, D.; Di Matteo, M.; Zaccardelli, M.; Campbell, C.G.; Woods, S. Total phenolics and condensed tannins in field pea (*Pisum sativum* L.) and grass pea (*Lathyrus sativus* L.). *Euphytica* **1998**, *101*, 97–102. [CrossRef]
22. Stanisavljević, N.; Jovanović, Z.; Čupić, T.; Lukić, J.; Miljuš Dukić, M.J.; Radović, S.; Mikić, A. Extractability of antioxidants from legume seed flour after cooking and in vitro gastrointestinal digestion in comparison with methanolic extraction of the unprocessed flour. *Int. J. Food Sci. Technol.* **2013**, *48*, 2096–2104.
23. Amarowicz, R.; Raab, B. Antioxidative activity of leguminous seed extracts evaluated by chemiluminescence methods. *Z. Naturforsch.* **1997**, *52*, 709–712. [CrossRef]
24. Naczk, M.; Shahidi, F. The effect of methanol-ammonia-water treatment on the content of phenolic acids of canola. *Food Chem.* **1989**, *31*, 159–164. [CrossRef]
25. Price, M.L.; van Scoyoc, S.; Butler, L.G. A critical evaluation of the vanillin reaction as an assay for tannin in sorghum grain. *J. Agric. Food Chem.* **1978**, *26*, 1214–1218. [CrossRef]
26. Re, R.; Pellegrini, N.; Proteggente, A.; Pannala, A.; Yang, M.; Rice-Evans, C. Antioxidant activity applying an improved ABTS radical cation decolorization assay. *Free Rad. Biol. Med.* **1999**, *26*, 1231–1237. [CrossRef]
27. Benzie, I.E.F.; Strain, J.J. Ferric reducing/antioxidant power assay: Direct measure of total antioxidant activity of biological fluids and modified version for simultaneous measurement of total antioxidant power and ascorbic acid concentration. *Methods Enzymol.* **1990**, *299*, 15–27.
28. Orak, H.-H.; Karamać, M.; Orak, A.; Amarowicz, R. Aantioxidant potential and phenolic compounds of some widely consumed Turkish white bean (*Phaseolus vulgaris* L.) varieties. *Pol. J. Food Nutr. Sci.* **2016**, *66*, 253–260. [CrossRef]
29. Fratianni, F.; Cardinale, F.; Cozzolino, A.; Granese, T.; Albanese, D.; Di Matteo, M.; Zaccardelli, M.; Coppola, R.; Nazzaro, F. Polyphenol composition and antioxidant activity of different grass pea (*Lathyrus sativus*), lentils (*Lens culinaris*), and chickpea (*Cicer arietinum*) ecotypes of the Campania region (Southern Italy). *J. Funct. Foods* **2014**, *7*, 551–557. [CrossRef]
30. Wiszniewska, A.; Piwowarczyk, B. Activity of selected components of antioxidant system in grass pea and yellow lupine protoplasts after enzymatic isolation. *Biotechnologia* **2015**, *96*, 285–292. [CrossRef]
31. Talukdar, D. Total flavonoids, phenolics, tannins and antioxidant activity in seeds of lentil and grass pea. *Int. J. Phytomed.* **2012**, *4*, 2096–2104.
32. Tamburino, R.; Guida, V.; Pacifico, S.; Rocco, M.; Zarelli, A.; Parente, A.; Di Maro, A. Nutritional values and radical scavenging capacities of grass pea (*Lathyrus sativus* L.) seeds in Valle Agricola district, Italy. *Austr. J. Crop. Sci.* **2012**, *6*, 149–156.
33. Starzyńska-Janiszewska, A.; Stodolak, B. Effect of inoculated lactic acid fermentation on antinutritional and antiradical properties of grass pea (*Lathyrus sativus* "Krab") flour. *Pol. J. Food Nutr. Sci.* **2011**, *61*, 245–249. [CrossRef]
34. Siddhuraju, P.; Becker, K. The antioxidant and free radical scavenging activities of processed cowpea (*Vigna unuguiculata* (L.) Walp.) seed extracts. *Food Chem.* **2007**, *101*, 10–19. [CrossRef]
35. Amarowicz, R.; Shahidi, F. Antioxidant activity of broad bean seed extract and its phenolic composition. *J. Funct. Foods* **2017**, *38*, 656–662. [CrossRef]
36. Amarowicz, R.; Shahidi, F. Antioxidant activity of faba bean extract and fractions thereof. *J. Food Bioact.* **2018**, *1*, 112–118. [CrossRef]
37. Amarowicz, R.; Estrella, I.; Hernández, T.; Troszyńska, A. Antioxidant activity of extract of adzuki bean and its fractions. *J. Food Lipids* **2008**, *15*, 119–136. [CrossRef]

38. Amarowicz, R.; Estrella, I.; Hernández, T.; Robredo, S.; Troszyńska, A.; Kosińska, A.; Pegg, R.B. Free radical-scavenging capacity, antioxidant activity, and phenolic composition of green lentil (*Lens culinaris*). *Food Chem.* **2010**, *121*, 705–711. [CrossRef]
39. Amarowicz, R.; Troszyńska, A.; Baryłko-Pikielna, N.; Shahidi, F. Polyphenolics extracts from legume seeds: Correlations between total antioxidant activity, total phenolics content, tannins content and astringency. *J. Food Lipids* **2004**, *11*, 278–286. [CrossRef]
40. Orak, H.H.; Karamać, M.; Amarowicz, R. Antioxidant activity of phenolic compounds of red bean (*Phaseolus vulgaris* L.). *Oxid. Commun.* **2015**, *38*, 67–76.

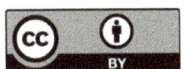 © 2018 by the authors. Licensee MDPI, Basel, Switzerland. This article is an open access article distributed under the terms and conditions of the Creative Commons Attribution (CC BY) license (http://creativecommons.org/licenses/by/4.0/).

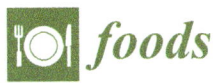

Article

Production, Quality, and Acceptance of *Tempeh* and White Bean *Tempeh* Burgers

Rayane J. Vital [1], Priscila Z. Bassinello [2,*], Quédma A. Cruz [3], Rosângela N. Carvalho [4], Júlia C. M. de Paiva [5] and Aline O. Colombo [6]

1. Faculty of Nutrition, Paulista University—UNIP, Goiânia 74845-090b, GO, Brazil; rayanevitalnutri@gmail.com
2. Department of Food Science, Embrapa Arroz e Feijão, Santo Antonio de Goiás 75375-000, GO, Brazil
3. Food Engineering School, Goias Federal University—UFG, Goiânia 74690-900, GO, Brazil; quedma.cruz@gmail.com
4. Grain and Byproducts Laboratory, Embrapa Arroz e Feijão, Santo Antonio de Goiás 75375-000, GO, Brazil; rosangela.carvalho@embrapa.br
5. Food Science and Technology School, Paulista University—UNIP, Goiânia 74845-090, GO, Brazil; judepaiva3108@gmail.com
6. Graduate Program on Food Science and Technology, Goias Federal University—UFG, Goiânia 74690-900, GO, Brazil; colomboaline@yahoo.com.br
* Correspondence: priscila.bassinello@embrapa.br; Tel.: +55-62-35332186

Received: 7 June 2018; Accepted: 25 August 2018; Published: 30 August 2018

Abstract: The food industry has been challenged to develop new healthy food products. *Tempeh*, originating in Indonesia and produced by fungal fermentation, would be an alternative healthy food for the Brazilian population. This study was designed to produce white bean (cv BRS Ártico) *tempeh* burger, to determine and compare its nutritional and sensory properties with conventional soybean-based *tempeh* burger. The production and the analyses of proximal composition and microbiological contamination were determined in the *tempeh*, following reference methods. For the sensory analysis, a nine-point hedonic scale test was performed with 82 untrained evaluators, and at the end, a question of purchase intent was answered. The results indicated significant differences in the nutritional value of the *tempehs*, which is justified by the difference in the composition of the raw materials used. The samples did not present a risk of microbiological contamination for consumption. The white bean *tempeh* burgers showed similar appearance and crispy consistency, but received lower scores for flavor, compared to the soybean burgers, probably due to their residual beany flavor. The beany flavor could be minimized by increasing the cooking time of the beans. White bean *tempeh* can be a good alternative for healthy eating, and its manufacture could promote the production of new products made from beans, giving a new focus to the Brazilians' traditional food. It is still necessary to improve the techniques of production and test new ingredients for the preparation of *tempeh* burgers to obtain higher acceptability.

Keywords: tempeh; *Phaseolus vulgaris* L.; nutritional value; sensory analysis; *Glycine max* L.

---

1. Introduction

The food industry has targeted healthy and diversified food for the development of new products in the market all over the world. The fermented food is one example of recent products demanded by a considerable population group whose interest in variability and new foods with functional, nutritional, and tasty attributes has increased lately [1]. *Tempeh* is a traditional Indonesian food, produced by fermentation of soybeans using *Rhizopus* species, having nutritional qualities and metabolic regulation functions [2]. It can also be produced from other substrates, such as beans, corn, rice, lentils, and barley.

Brazil, being one of the largest producers, consumers and holders of technologies for bean production, could engage in this promising field by encouraging research on beans [3].

Phaseolus vulgaris L. (common beans) is one of the primary sources of protein and one of the essential foods for the Brazilian population. It presents an average protein content of 28% and has all the essential amino acids in its composition; it is rich in lysine, but limiting in sulfur amino acids—methionine and cysteine [4]. Although there is a regional preference for a specific type of beans, those from the *Carioca* group are the 16 most cultivated in Brazil, representing 70% of the national consumption, cultivar Pérola being the most consumed [5]. There is also a growing potential for types of beans with different characteristics of color, shape, and size, attracting gourmet gastronomy for different culinary preparations and in the food industry, not only as the traditional cooked beans [6]. Fermentation of leguminous seeds as beans has several advantages, since it reduces non-nutritional factors, improves nutrient digestibility, reduces allergenicity, activates antioxidant activity, and the concentration of phenolic compounds can be increased during the fermentation process, in addition to being associated with the reduction of chronic diseases risk. Therefore, there is a growing interest in promoting the production of fermented leguminous seeds [7].

The 68th United Nations General Assembly declared 2016 the International Year of Pulses to raise public awareness of the nutritional benefits, sustainable production, food security, nutrition, creating an opportunity to encourage better utilization of plant proteins, crop rotation and the trade of "pulses" [8]. In this context, there are countries in Africa and Asia, such as Indonesia and India, where *tempeh*, due to its nutritional and sensory properties and versatility in the preparation in pure form or as an ingredient in a number of other food preparations (hamburgers—"green meat", vegetarian products, lyophilized or roasted *tempeh* flour for biscuits), has been stimulated in public policies, as an alternative in the multimixtures to fight the malnutrition of deprived populations, especially in mothers and children undergoing weaning [9].

The objective of this work was to develop *tempeh* and *tempeh* burgers from white beans (cv BRS Arctic) without tegument by solid fermentation and to compare their nutritional and sensorial characteristics with conventional soybean *tempeh* burgers.

2. Materials and Methods

2.1. Acquisition of the Material

Beans of cultivars BRS Arctic and conventional soybeans BRS 284 used in this study were from the 2015 harvest season at Fazenda Capivara, Embrapa Arroz e Feijão/GO/Brazil. The *Rhizopus oligosporus* strain was purchased from the Tropical Cultures Collection of André Tosello Research and Technology Foundation, Campinas/SP. Samples of soybean tempehs, commercial products of the same lot, were purchased from Totale Tempeh manufacturer at Rezende/RJ/Brazil and used as reference.

2.2. Raw Material Preparation

Dry beans and soybeans were homogenized, sorted manually, and only the whole and healthy ones were selected, placed in polyethylene bags, and stored in a cold room until use.

2.3. Rhizopus oligosporus Multiplication

Rhizopus oligosporus strains were transferred to Petri dishes with PDA (Potato Dextrose Agar) medium for increased spore production. After mycelial growth and spore formation, the surface of each plate was scraped with a platinum handle and the mycelium transferred to an Erlenmeyer flask containing 100 mL of sterile distilled water and counting performed in the Neubauer chamber, as reported by Miyaoka [10]. To determine the ideal culture medium for inoculum production, the *Rhizopus* strain was seeded in Petri dishes containing the following media: Potato Agar Dextrose (PDA), PDA + rice flour, PDA + bean flour, PDA + 50% rice flour + 50% bean flour. The autoclaved culture media were inoculated in a laminar flow chamber and incubated in an oven at 30 °C for 48 h. The medium presenting the best fungus development was chosen for inoculum preparation.

2.4. Spore Counting

Spore counts were performed using the Neubauer chamber (Global Trade, Double Improved—BSN 020; Hatfield, PA) where 0.2 mL of the suspension was homogenized and transferred to a test tube and 0.6 ml of 0.2% trypan blue dye was added. A 0.5 mL aliquot was then placed on a cover plate for spore counting under the microscope. For calculation of number of cells/mL, Equation (1) was used:

Number of cells/mL = (total number of cells × dilution factor × 10,000)/number of quadrants counted (1)

2.5. Inoculum Preparation

For the production of the flour inoculum, 100 g of type 1 rice were grounded and sieved on a BERTEL® vibrating sieve (Caieiras, SP, Brazil) using 200 mesh sieves. The flour was placed in glass containers with metal lid, sterilized, and cooled at room temperature. Twenty milliliters of the inoculum was inoculated into each vessel and incubated in an oven at 30 °C for 5 days. After this period, the containers were refrigerated and used for up to 30 days.

2.6. Tempeh Production

Tempehs were prepared following the methodology used by Starzynska-Janiszewska et al. [11]. Two hundred grams of beans were cleaned in running water, submerged in 1000 mL of sterilized water at room temperature for hydration/maceration with the addition of 20 mL of commercial alcohol vinegar containing acetic acid (5%) for 20 h. For the removal of surface water, beans were dried on paper towels at room temperature and the tegument removed manually. Heat treatment was performed by conditioning the beans in beakers capped with laminated paper, autoclaving them for 15 min at 121 °C, and then draining them and cooling at room temperature. After those procedures, beans were placed in polyethylene bags and inoculated with 20 g of the inoculum previously produced with rice flour and strain of *Rhizopus oligosporus*. The bags were sealed and small holes were made with a fork to allow the contact of the fungus with oxygen. Finally, beans were incubated in an oven at 30 °C and visually monitored to follow up on the development of the mycelium (about 30 h) (Figure 1).

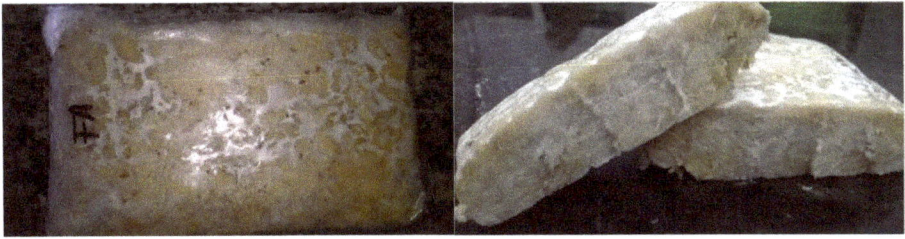

Figure 1. *Tempeh* of white beans after mycelium total development.

2.7. Analytical Determinations

White bean and soybean *tempehs* samples were dehydrated by lyophilization in a LIOTOP® L101 lyophilizer equipment (São Carlos, SP, Brazil) for 48 h until all material was completely dehydrated. The nutritional characterization was performed by official methods according to the Association of Official Analytical Chemists (AOAC) 2010 [12]. The moisture content was determined by oven-drying at 105 °C until constant weight; the ash content was evaluated by the gravimetric method of incineration in a muffle oven at 500 °C; the lipid content was determined by continuous extraction in a Soxhlet apparatus using ethyl ether as solvent; the total nitrogen content was obtained by the micro-Kjeldahl method using the factor 6.25 for conversion into protein; the total dietary fiber was analyzed by the gravimetric-enzymatic method established by AOAC 2005 [13] and adapted by Embrapa Agroindústria de Alimentos [14], and the carbohydrate content was calculated by difference, as provided by the Resolution of the Collegiate Board of Directors (RDC) No. 360, December 2, 200,315 by Equation (2):

$$\% \text{ carbohydrate} = 100 - (\% \text{ ash} + \% \text{ protein} + \% \text{ lipid} + \% \text{fiber}) \qquad (2)$$

The energy value of the product was estimated using Atwater conversion factors of 4 kcal/g for protein and carbohydrate and 9 kcal/g for lipid [15].

2.8. Microbiological Analysis

The presence of the following microorganisms in the ready-made *tempehs* was analyzed as follows: Coliforms, Staphylococcus positive coagulase and *Salmonella* sp. at 45 °C. The microbiological protocol followed the methodology established by the Compendium of Methods for the Microbiological Examination of Foods [16]. For all analyzed microorganisms, a control test (incubation of the culture medium in a petri dish, without inoculation) was performed to verify the innocuity.

2.9. Hamburgers Preparation

For the sensorial analysis, hamburgers were chosen as an alternative for using *tempeh*, because that food is easy to handle and popular among the surveyed public. The same additional ingredients and amounts (Table 1) were used in the formulation of both *tempehs*. They were homogenized in a Mondial® culinary multiprocessor (Brasília, DF, Brazil), manually molded, and grilled in a nonstick frying pan with olive oil until golden brown on both sides. Each 100 g of *tempeh* yielded an average of 11 small burgers.

Table 1. Additional ingredients for 100 g *tempeh* burger preparation.

Ingredients	Amount
Salt	2 g
Pepper	2 g
Dehydrated onion	3 g
Dehydrated garlic	3 g
Dehydrated parsley	4 g
Dehydrated green onions	4 g
Olive oil	50 mL

2.10. Tempeh Burgers Sensory Evaluation

Tempeh burgers were evaluated by 82 nontrained participants for their appearance, aroma, flavor, and overall impression, using a nine-point hedonic scale (9—I liked very much, 8—I liked it a lot, 7—I liked it moderately, 6—I liked it slightly, 5—I did not like it or disliked, 4—I disliked it slightly, 3—I Disliked it moderately, 2—I did not like it much and 1—I did not like it very much). The tasters were also asked about their purchase intent (I would definitely buy this product, I would probably buy this product, I'm not sure if I would buy this product, I probably would not buy this product, I certainly would not buy this product). The participants were students from the Department of Pharmacy of the Metropolitan College of Anápolis—GO, employees of the Embrapa Rice and Beans Research Center and students from the Federal University of Goiás. They were over 18-year-old nonsmokers, healthy nonpregnant women and men, randomly selected. The participants filled out a Term of free consent and the Consolidated view of the research ethics committee of the Federal University of Goiás, and before receiving the samples were instructed how they should conduct the test. The sensorial analysis was carried out in the Food Technology Laboratory at the Metropolitan College of Anápolis, GO and in the Experimental Kitchen Laboratory at Embrapa Rice and Beans Research Center, Santo Antônio de Goiás, GO. The laboratories have sensory booths for analysis, as well as adequate lighting and kitchen support.

Two samples were made available, the first one being of white bean *tempeh* and the second of soybean *tempeh*. A questionnaire was distributed along with a glass of water and samples served in disposable dishes. The project was submitted to the evaluation and approval of the Research Ethics Committee of the Federal University of Goiás under protocol No. 60631116.6.0000.5083.

2.11. Statistical Analysis

Results were analyzed by ANOVA and F test using SISVAR® software, followed by independent 2 group *t* test using software-R ($p < 0.05$) for comparison of the mean values obtained in the different treatments. For sensory evaluation of mean descriptive values, Tukey test ($p < 0.05$) was applied instead.

3. Results and Discussion

3.1. Microbiological Analysis

Hygienic-sanitary care during the food manufacturing process is a preventive measure of microbiological contamination and has been a concern of the sanitary inspection agencies. All food must have its quality proven by tests that justify its innocuity [17]. After the production of the *tempehs*, the microbial investigation of the samples was carried out and the results found are expressed in Table 2.

Table 2. Evaluation of the microbiological contamination of *tempehs*.

Identification	Coliforms 45 °C/g	Staph. Positive Coag./g	*Salmonella* sp./25 g
White bean *Tempeh*	≤10 CFU	≤10 CFU	Absence in 25 g
Soybean *Tempeh*	≤10 CFU	≤10 CFU	Absence in 25 g
Microbiological Reference Limits *	10^2 CFU/g	10^2 CFU/g	Absence in 25 g

* Source: Adapted from Resolution of the Collegiate Board of Directors (RDC) No. 12, 2 January 2001, for fermented foods.

From the data obtained, it can be observed that results for the three microorganisms studied were within the standards established by RDC No. 12, which includes values for Colony-Forming Units (CFU) in fermented foods, thus proving that there was no significant growth of typical colonies of bacteria that could affect the microbiological quality of the product, making *tempeh* safe for consumption. Autoclaving and acidification of the medium, steps used in this study, are useful techniques to control *tempeh* contaminating agents, but it is worth mentioning that good manufacturing practices also contribute to the absence of pathogenic bacteria, as well as storage conditions.

3.2. Nutritional Characterization

The nutritional value of the *tempehs* is naturally different due to the composition of the raw material (Table 3).

Table 3. Proximal composition * and calories content of white bean and soybean *tempehs*.

Identification	Moisture (%)	Ash (g/100 g)	Lipid (g/100 g)	Protein (g/100 g)	CHO (g/100 g)	Kcal/100 g
White bean *tempeh*	3.94 ± 0.10 [a]	2.40 ± 0.08 [a]	1.29 ± 0.04 [b]	23.34 ± 0.21 [b]	55.45 [a]	326.77 [b]
Soybean *tempeh*	2.57 ± 0.12 [b]	2.03 ± 0.01 [b]	24.88 ± 0.30 [a]	43.74 ± 0.28 [a]	10.39 [b]	440.44 [a]

* Means from three determinations ± standard deviation followed by the same lowercase letter in the same column do not differ by the *t*-test at 5% significance ($p < 0.05$).

It is important to emphasize the significant difference observed in the lipid analyses, where the soybean *tempeh* presented 24.88 g/100 g, while that of white bean 1.29 g/100 g, and this difference impacts and explains the significantly different caloric values of both *tempehs*. The white bean *tempeh* sample showed fewer calories because of the lower lipid and intermediate protein contents compared to the soybean *tempeh*. According to Astuti et al. [18], the protein content of soybean *tempehs* and soybeans are practically the same. Due to the action of the protease enzyme produced by the fungus during fermentation, the soluble protein content increases markedly. The soluble nitrogen content in unfermented soybeans is 3.5 mg/g, compared to 8.7 mg/g in *tempehs*. Beans are an excellent food, providing essential nutrients, such as iron and calcium, carbohydrates, and fibers. They are the primary source of protein for the Brazilian low-income population, but the digestibility of these proteins is relatively low. According to Mesquita et al. (2007), the protein value of the white bean *tempeh* does not increase significantly after fermentation, and the value here was 23.34 g/100 g [19]. However, it is reported in the literature that *Rhizopus* uses amino acids as a source of nitrogen for its growth. This might suggest that the total amino acid content decreases, but free amino acids increase, making white bean *tempeh* protein probably more digestible than cooked beans.

3.3. Total Food Fiber

Regarding total fiber content, white bean and soybean *tempehs* showed no significant difference, except for the insoluble fiber fraction (Table 4).

Table 4. Dietary fiber fractions in white bean and soybean *tempehs* *.

Identification	Soluble Dietary Fiber (g/100 g)	Insoluble Dietary Fiber (g/100 g)	Total Dietary Fiber (g/100 g)
White bean *Tempeh*	4.11 [a]	13.40 [b]	17.52 [a]
Soybean *Tempeh*	2.18 [a]	16.80 [a]	18.96 [a]

* Same lowercase letters in the same column do not differ by the *t*-test at 5% significance ($p < 0.05$).

According to FAO/WHO, an adult individual needs about 25 grams of fiber per day, which makes *tempeh* products interesting for fiber supply, and they may also act in the control of intestinal transit and the treatment of comorbidities such as obesity.

4. Sensory Analysis

Hamburgers of both *tempehs* presented a firm and consistent shape, similar appearance, pleasant odor, a brownish crust and a certain degree of crunchiness (Figure 2).

For appearance, 68.29% of the participants liked the white bean *tempeh* burger, and 23.17% liked it very much. Not very dissenting results were obtained for the soy burger, where 74.39% of the participants reported liking the appearance of the product, and 28% liked it very much. Among these, 16 evaluators disliked the white bean *tempeh* hamburger and eight, the soy one. The aesthetic parameter is one of the central questions taken into account by the consumer when assessing the safety of food, which incorporates a different concept of food safety, taking into account technical concepts such as odor, nutritional value, and appearance. The appearance of the *tempeh* burgers was considered to be nice, resembling chicken burgers.

For flavor, 47.56% of the participants reported liking the white bean *tempeh* burger, with only 6% of the individuals showing a great liking for the product; a very different result for the soy *tempeh* hamburger, where 68.29% liked the product at different intensities, and 24.39% showed great liking. Of the total participants, 34.15% disliked the white bean *tempeh* burger and 20.73% the soy one. This can be explained by the fact that the aroma of the bean is not part of the olfactory memory linked to the aroma of hamburgers. When one imagines or visualizes a food, the aroma, and the flavor are automatically sought in the subconscious, and when one tastes it one expects an aroma that is already similar to the known [20]. The storage conditions of the beans and even the ready-made *tempeh* may have resulted in the loss of quality causing the off flavor due to the oxidation of the beans' unsaturated fatty acids. The unpleasant taste and odor in the soy products are attributed to the action of lipoxygenase enzymes, which form hydroperoxides from polyunsaturated fatty acids [21].

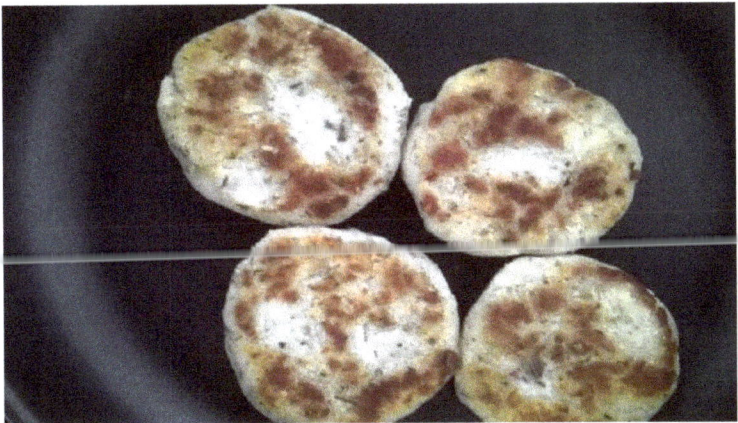

Figure 2. White bean *tempeh* burger.

For flavor evaluation, 39.02% of the participants said they liked the white bean *tempeh* burger, and 53% liked the soy one. Of the total participants, 35 of them disliked the white bean *tempeh* burger, and only 17 disliked the soybean. The same considerations regarding aroma are applied to flavor since this attribute is a mixture of olfactory, gustatory, and tactile sensations. There were reports of the presence of a residual flavor in both burgers. The remaining taste in the mouth sometime after the food has been swallowed seems to be more noticeable in the white bean burger. The autoxidation of the fatty acids present in the soybean generates several classes of volatile compounds, which contribute to the residual taste of 'green grass'. One hypothesis for the low acceptance of the soy and white bean *tempeh* burgers would be their manufacturing process, which had a shorter cooking time compared to soybeans and home-cooked beans. The overall impression (Table 5) depicts a collection of prejudged elements that define the appraiser's appreciation of the product as a whole. In this case, the soy *tempeh* burger obtained higher scores than the white bean *tempeh* one, presenting a higher performance in all attributes.

Table 5. Overall scores of the sensorial analysis of white bean and soybean *tempeh* burgers *.

Identification	Appearance	Aroma	Flavor	Overall Impression
White bean *tempeh*	6.22 [a]	4.00 [b]	3.55 [b]	5.10 [b]
Soybean *tempeh*	6.93 [a]	6.54 [a]	6.35 [a]	6.40 [a]

* Same lowercase letters in the same column do not differ by the Tukey test at 5% significance ($p < 0.05$).

In general, the soybean burger had a higher average score for all attributes, but there was no significant difference in appearance, demonstrating that both burgers were similar. Figure 3 shows that the buying intention for the soy *tempeh* burger was higher than that for the white bean *tempeh* burger, which is consistent with the attributes previously analyzed.

Burgers can be one of several options for the use of *tempeh*. The low purchase intent may be associated with the fact that the consumers connect the hamburger with characteristics of succulence, meat flavor, frying smell, and darker color. Shurtleff et al. [22], in the mid-1980s, mentioned that soybean burgers were used in campaigns in Europe to promote the consumption of soy-based products as a beef substitute and as a healthy food. When faced with the bean samples, the expectation created for the consumption of this food is dissolved by the difference from traditional hamburgers.

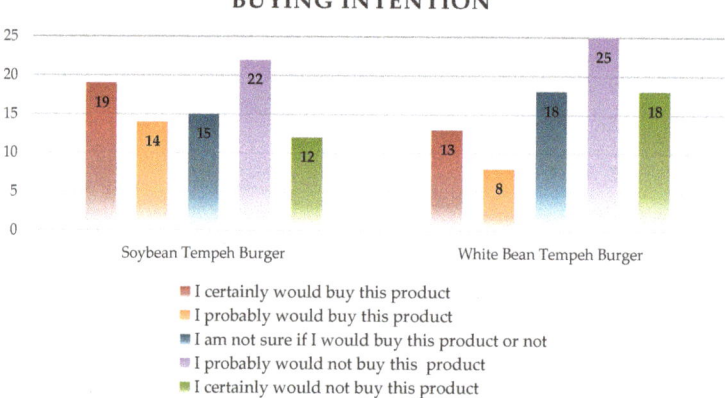

Figure 3. Purchase intention for the *tempeh* burger.

5. Conclusions

White bean *tempeh* is an innovative food; it has good nutritional value, with a considerable amount of protein; may be an alternative and eventually an option for meat, and can be consumed by vegetarians and sympathizers. It also has a high content of carbohydrates, calories, and a good source of fibers, being an excellent product for energy intake, and if inserted in a balanced diet, it may act as intestinal regulator. The soybean *tempeh* burger showed higher scores in all attributes evaluated in the sensory analysis, demonstrating the need for further research to either improve *tempeh* production techniques and to use other ingredients for the preparation of hamburgers or other *tempeh* products to provide greater acceptance of this new product. White bean *tempeh* could be a good alternative for healthy eating, but its recommendation should be based on scientific studies which demonstrate its beneficial effects. Continuous scientific research is necessary to identify beneficial components, their mechanisms of action, function, nutritional aspects. The production of legume-based *tempeh* can promote the creation of new products made from common beans, giving an alternative to the traditional Brazilian food.

Finally, we believe that this study has some potential social and economic impacts such as the contribution to the advancement of scientific knowledge regarding the pioneering process of manufacturing *tempeh* in Brazil; it gives nutritionists the opportunity to explore the versatility of common beans in gastronomy; improves the bean production chain as well as the small farmer's techniques, and gives them the opportunity to explore different common bean cultivars.

Author Contributions: Conceptualization, P.Z.B.; Methodology, A.O.C.; Formal Analysis, R.J.V. and Q.A.C.; Investigation, P.Z.B. and R.J.V.; Resources, P.Z.B. and R.N.C.; Data Curation, R.J.V.; Writing-Original Draft Preparation, R.J.V.; Writing-Review & Editing, P.Z.B. and J.C.M.d.P.; Visualization, P.Z.B.; Supervision, P.Z.B. and A.O.C.; Project Administration, P.Z.B.; Funding Acquisition, P.Z.B.

Funding: This research was funded by Embrapa and by a CNPq scholarship.

Acknowledgments: The authors thank the National Council for Scientific and Technological Development (CNPq), Embrapa Rice and Beans Research Center for the scientific/financial support and the Grain and Byproducts Laboratory together with its staff and the Metropolitan College of Anápolis-GO.

Conflicts of Interest: The authors declare that there is no conflict of interest.

References

1. Cruz, I.L. Desenvolvimento de um Inóculo Seguro, Eficiente e Padronizado para a Produção de Tempeh em Pequena Escala a Partir de Diferentes Leguminosas. Master's Thesis, Universidade de Lisboa, Lisboa, Portugal, 2014.

2. Nakajima, N.; Nozaki, N.; Ishihara, K.; Ishikawa, A.; Tsuji, H. Analysis of isoflavone content in *tempeh*, a fermented soybean, and preparation of a new isoflavone-enriched tempeh. *J. Biosci. Bioeng.* **2005**, *100*, 685–687. [CrossRef] [PubMed]
3. Krisnawati, A.; Adie, M.M. Selection of soybean genotypes by seed size and its prospects for industrial raw material in Indonesia. *Procedia Food. Sci.* **2015**, *3*, 355–363. [CrossRef]
4. Carvalho, A.V.; Bassinello, P.Z.; Mattietto, R.A.; Carvalho, R.N.; Rios, A.O.; Seccadio, L.L. Processamento e caracterização de snack extrudado a partir de farinhas de quirera de arroz e de bandinha de feijão. *Braz. J. Food. Technol.* **2012**, *15*, 72–83. [CrossRef]
5. Vanier, N.L. Armazenamento de Cultivares de Feijão e seus Efeitos na Qualidade Tecnológica dos grãos e nas Propriedades do Amido. Master's Thesis, Universidade Federal de Pelotas, Pelotas, Brazil, 2012.
6. Souza, T.L.P.O.; Pereira, H.S.; Faria, L.C.; Wendland, A.; Cost, J.G.C.; Abreu, Â.F.B.; (Embrapa Arroz e Feijão, Santo Antônio de Goiás, Goiás, Brasil). Personal communication, 2010.
7. Limón, R.I.; Peñas, E.; Torino, M.I.; Martínez-Villaluenga, C.; Dueñas, M.; Frias, J. Fermentation enhances the content of bioactive compounds in kidney bean extracts. *Food. Chem.* **2015**, *172*, 343–352. [CrossRef] [PubMed]
8. FAO (Food and Agriculture Organization of the United Nations). International Year of Pulses. 2016. Available online: http://www.un.org/en/ga/search/viewdoc.asp?symbol=A/RES/68/231&referer=http://www.un.org/en/events/observances/years.shtml&Lang=E (accessed on 25 February 2016).
9. Scrimshaw, N.S.; Wallerstein, M.B. *Nutrition Policy Implementation: Issuesand Experience*; Springer Science & Business Media: Berlin, Germany, 2012.
10. Miyaoaka, M.F. Avaliação do Potencial dos Fungos do gênero *Rhizopus* spp. na Produção de Substâncias Bioativas com Ação Antioxidante Utilizando Diferentes Substratos. Master's Thesis, Universidade Federal do Paraná, Setor de Tecnologia, Pelotas, Brazil, 2012.
11. Starzyńska-Janiszewska, A.; Stodolak, B.; Mickowska, B. Effect of controlled lactic acid fermentation on selected bioactive and nutritional parameters of tempeh obtained from unhulled common bean (*Phaseolus vulgaris*) seeds. *J. Sci. Food. Agric.* **2014**, *94*, 359–366. [CrossRef] [PubMed]
12. Association of Official Analytical Chemists. *Official Methods of Analysis*, 19th ed.; AOAC: Washington, DC, USA, 2010.
13. Association of Official Analytical Chemists. *Official Methods of Analysis of the Association Analytical Chemists*, 18th ed.; AOAC: Gaithersburg, MD, USA, 2005.
14. Freitas, S.C.; Carvalho, P.G.B.; Tupinambá, D.D.; Koakuzu, S.N.; Carvalho, A.V.; (Embrapa Arroz e Feijão, Santo Antônio de Goiás, Goiás, Brasil). Personal communication, 2008.
15. MERRIL, A.L.; WATT, B.K. *Energy Value of Foods: Basis and Derivation*; United States Department of Agriculture: Washington, DC, USA, 1973.
16. American Public Health Association. *Compendium of Methods for the Microbiological Examination for Foods*, 4th ed.; American Public Health Association: Washington, DC, USA, 2001.
17. Griese, S.E.; Fleischauer, A.T.; Macfarquhar, J.K.; Moore, Z.; Harrelson, C.; Valiani, A. Gastroenteritis Outbreak Associated with Unpasteurized *Tempeh*, North Carolina, USA. *Emerg. Infect. Dis.* **2013**, *19*, 1514–1517. [CrossRef] [PubMed]
18. Astuti, M.; Meliala, A.; Dalais, F.S.; Wahlqvist, M.L. Tempeh, a nutritious and healthy food from Indonesia. *Asia Pac. J. Clin. Nutr.* **2000**, *9*, 322–325. [CrossRef] [PubMed]
19. Mesquita, F.R.; Corrêa, A.D.; Abreu, C.M.P.; Lima, R.A.Z.; Abreu, A.F.B. Linhagens de feijão (*Phaseolus vulgaris* L.): Composição química e digestibilidade protéica. *Cienc. Agrotecnol.* **2007**, *31*, 1114–1121. [CrossRef]
20. Teixeira, L.V. Análise sensorial na indústria de alimentos. *Revista do Instituto de Laticínios Cândido Tostes* **2009**, *64*, 12–21.
21. Ciabotti, S.; Barcelos, M.F.P.; Pinheiro, A.C.M.; Clemente, P.R.; Lima, M.A.C. Características sensoriais e físicas de extratos e tofus de soja comum processada termicamente e livre de lipoxigenase. *Ciênc. Technol. Aliment.* **2007**, *27*, 643–648. [CrossRef]
22. Shurtleff, W.; Aoyagi, A. *The Book of Tempeh*, 2nd ed.; Soyinfo Center: Lafayette, CA, USA, 1979.

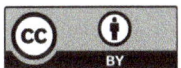

© 2018 by the authors. Licensee MDPI, Basel, Switzerland. This article is an open access article distributed under the terms and conditions of the Creative Commons Attribution (CC BY) license (http://creativecommons.org/licenses/by/4.0/).

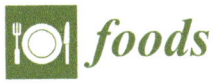

Article

Nutritional Characterization of *Prosopis laevigata* Legume Tree (Mesquite) Seed Flour and the Effect of Extrusion Cooking on its Bioactive Components

Luis Díaz-Batalla [1,2], Juan P. Hernández-Uribe [3], Roberto Gutiérrez-Dorado [4], Alejandro Téllez-Jurado [5], Javier Castro-Rosas [1], Rogelio Pérez-Cadena [5] and Carlos A. Gómez-Aldapa [1,*]

1. Área Académica de Química, Universidad Autónoma del Estado de Hidalgo, Carretera Pachuca-Tulancingo Km 4.5, Mineral de la Reforma, C.P. 42184 Hidalgo, Mexico; ldiaz@upfim.edu.mx (L.D.-B.); jcastro@uaeh.edu.mx (J.C.-R.)
2. Ingeniería Agroindustrial, Universidad Politécnica de Francisco I. Madero, Tepatepec, C.P. 42660 Hidalgo, Mexico
3. Instituto de Ciencias Agropecuarias, Universidad Autónoma del Estado de Hidalgo, Av. Universidad Km 1, Rancho Universitario, Tulancingo de Bravo, C.P. 43600 Hidalgo, Mexico; hdezspark@hotmail.com
4. Facultad de Ciencias Químico Biológicas, Universidad Autónoma de Sinaloa, Ciudad Universitaria, Culiacan, C.P. 80040 Sinaloa, Mexico; robe399@hotmail.com
5. Departamento de Biotecnología, Universidad Politécnica de Pachuca, Zempoala, C.P. 43830 Hidalgo, Mexico; alito@upp.edu.mx (A.T.-J.); rpcadena1904@gmail.com (R.P.-C.)
* Correspondence: cgomeza@uaeh.edu.mx; Tel.: +52-771-717-2000 (ext. 2518)

Received: 8 July 2018; Accepted: 25 July 2018; Published: 1 August 2018

Abstract: Mesquite (*Prosopis laevigata*) is a legume tree widely distributed in Aridoamerica. The mature fruit of this legume is a pod, which is currently underutilized and has high nutritional potential. In the present work, mesquite seed flour is described in terms of its nutritional value, as well as the effect of extrusion cooking on its bioactive components. Mesquite seed flour is rich in fiber (7.73 g/100 g) and protein (36.51 g/100 g), with valine as the only limiting amino acid. Total phenolic compound contents in raw and extruded seed flour were 6.68 and 6.46 mg of gallic acid equivalents/g (mg GAE/g), respectively. 2-2-Diphenyl-1-picrylhydrazyl (DPPH) radical scavenging capacity values in raw and extruded seed flour were 9.11 and 9.32 mg of ascorbic acid equivalent/g (mg AAE/g), respectively. The absorbance at 290 nm, as an indicator of generation of Maillard reaction product (MRP), was the same for raw and extruded samples. Apigenin was the only flavonoid found in mesquite seed flour (41.6 mg/kg) and was stable in the extrusion process. The water absorption index (WAI) and water solubility index (WSI) were changed significantly during extrusion. The expansion of mesquite seed flour extrudates was null due to the high protein and fiber content in the sample. Extrusion cooking of mesquite seed flour is a useful form of technology for the industrialization of this underutilized and nutritionally valuable legume.

Keywords: mesquite; *Prosopis laevigata*; extrusion; phenolic compounds; radical scavenging capacity; apigenin

1. Introduction

Legumes have been an essential part of the human diet for centuries, with a major role in global food security, environmental challenges, and healthy diets [1]. Legumes have mastered symbiotic nitrogen fixation, leading to significant advantages for agricultural sustainability; however, they contribute to just a small portion of staple foods worldwide compared with cereals [2]. A shift in land use towards grain legumes would substantially lower the carbon footprint of the production of protein for human consumption [2]. Consumption of legumes seeds contributes to reduced risk of mortality because of their benefits against major chronic diseases and their risk factors due to their bioactive components [3,4]. Orphan crops are minor crops with regional importance that have been largely neglected by researchers and industry due to limited economic importance in the global market [2]. Orphan food legumes are usually grown in arid regions, often on marginal land unsuitable for major crop species. They have heat- and drought-tolerant traits and high nutritional value [2,4]. Wild and underutilized legumes with high nutraceutical value should be explored for overcoming protein energy malnutrition. The presence of anti-nutrients in legume seeds might not be an impediment, as proper processing methods can make them edible for a safe use [5]. Extrusion cooking technology is a high-temperature, short, and versatile food operation that converts agricultural raw materials into fully cooked and shelf-stable food products with enhanced nutritional attributes [6]. Legume extrusion cooking eliminates anti-nutritional factors and improves protein digestibility at a cost lower than other cooking systems [6,7]. Legumes could be included as protein sources in the extrusion process to formulate nutritionally enhanced functional food products [6].

The genus *Prosopis* is comprised of a group of nitrogen-fixing trees belonging to the Fabaceae family distributed in arid and semiarid regions of Asia, Africa, and America. *Prosopis* species were a major staple food for indigenous peoples in arid regions of America before the arrival of Europeans [8]. The mature fruit of the genus *Prosopis* is an indehiscent pod formed of an exocarp, a developed mesocarp, and a woody endocarp which protects the seed [8]. Pod flour of *Prosopis* is a versatile ingredient with high potential for the food industry. It is rich in protein, sugars, and fiber, and is gluten-free [8–10]. Pods of the *Prosopis* species have been reported as a source of bioactive compounds with antioxidant, inflammatory, and antihypertensive activities [8,11–13]. Seed flour of *Prosopis alba* showed high levels of proteins, minerals, fiber, and phenolic compounds, mainly flavones, with low content of total carbohydrates and fats [9,14]. Pod flour of *Prosopis laevigata* is a good source of lysine, sulfur-containing amino acids, and total phenolic compounds, with higher radical scavenging capacity than soybeans and common beans [15]. Thermal treatment of *P. laevigata* flours (for example in a baking process) increases the apparent total phenolic compound content and radical scavenging capacity, an effect associated with the generation of Maillard reaction products (MRPs) [15]. In order to increase the description of the nutritional value of the *Prosopis* genera, and explore technological options for its processing, in the present work the seed flour of the specie *P. laevigata*, widely distributed in Aridoamerica, is described in its nutritional value, and the bioactive compounds content is analyzed in raw and extruded mesquite seed flour.

2. Materials and Methods

2.1. Chemicals

Gallic acid, 2-2-diphenyl-1-picrylhydrazyl (DPPH), Folin–Ciocalteu's phenol reagent, daidzein, genistein, myricetin, quercetina, kaempferol, and apigenin were from Sigma (St. Louis, MO, USA).

2.2. Plant Material and Preparation of Mesquite Seed Flour

Dry mature pods were collected from trees of *P. laevigata* at the experimental field of the Universidad Politécnica de Francisco I. Madero in the semiarid region of the Mezquital Valley in Hidalgo, Mexico. Collected yellow-brown mature pods were ground using a 900-W blender (Nutribullet, Los Angeles, CA, USA). Milled pods was sieved in a 30 mesh, retaining the intact endocarp. The intact endocarp was submitted to a second milling process, producing seed flour which passed through an 80 mesh and the retained brans.

2.3. Seed Flour Chemical Composition

Crude fat, protein, moisture, fiber, and ash contents of seed flour were determined according to the procedures described in the Association of Official Analytical Chemists (AOAC), methods 920.39, 992.15, 925.09, 991.43, and 923.03, respectively [16].

2.4. Seed Flour Amino Acid Profile

The amino acid content in raw flour was analyzed after hydrolysis with 6 N HCl, using a cation exchange separation column (LCA K06/Na, 4.6 × 150 mm; Sykam GmbH, Eresing, Germany) with ninhydrin postcolumn derivatization, in an amino acid analyzer (Sykam GmbH, Eresing, Germany) [15]. The same method was used for sulfur-containing amino acids, using performic acid oxidation before hydrolysis [17]. Tryptophan was determined at 600 nm, after enzymatic hydrolysis with papain, and reaction with p-dimethylaminobenzaldehyde [18].

2.5. Seed Flour Extrusion

Seed flour was conditioned with purified water to obtain a moisture content of 16%. Seed flour was extruded in single screw extruder (Brabender 19/25DN, Duisburg, Germany) equipped with a 19-mm diameter and 3:1 compression ratio screw, working at 170 rpm. Barrel temperatures were 80, 100, 120, and 150 °C for zones 1, 2, 3, and 4, respectively. Feeder rate was set at 30 rpm and the diameter of the exit die was 3 mm. Seed flour extrudate was dried and ground until it passed through 80 mesh.

2.6. Preparation of Extracts

Raw seed flour and extruded seed flour were extracted with aqueous ethanol [15]. Samples of 100 mg were extracted with one milliliter of 40% ethanol in water (v/v) and centrifuged at 12,000 rpm/10 min. The extract was removed and the extraction process was done again with the residual pellet. Both extracts were mixed and diluted with 40% ethanol to obtain a final volume of 25 mL. These extracts were used for total phenolic compound content, radical scavenging capacity, and absorbance at 290 nm. For flavonoids, a replicate was prepared for each obtained extract and they were submitted to HCl hydrolysis with ethyl acetate aglycone recovery [19]. The ethyl acetate was evaporated at 45 °C and the residue was diluted in absolute ethanol to obtain a final volume of 2 mL.

2.7. Total Phenolic Compounds

Total phenolic compounds content was determined in raw and extruded seed flour extracts by the Folin–Ciocalteu reagent method [11]. The absorbance was measured at 760 nm and the results were expressed as mg of gallic acid equivalents/g (mg GAE/g) of dry weight.

2.8. DPPH Radical Scavenging Capacity

The radical scavenging capacity of raw and extruded seed flour extracts was determined using the DPPH synthetic radical method [11]. The absorbance was measured at 515 nm and the results were expressed as mg of ascorbic acid equivalent/g (mg AAE/g) of dry weight.

2.9. Ultraviolet Analysis of Maillard Reaction Products (MRPs)

Analysis of MRPs in extracts of raw and extruded flours was performed using the spectrophotometric method reported by Yu et al. [20]. Appropriate dilutions of extracts were scanned from 240 to 320 nm using an ultraviolet-visible (UV-VIS) spectrophotometer (Genesys 10 S, Thermo Scientific, Waltham, MA, USA). The presence of MRP was evidenced by the increase in the UV absorbance at 290 nm.

2.10. Flavonoids

The flavonoid content was determined by reversed-phase high-performance liquid chromatography (RP-HPLC) using a Dionex Ultimate 3000-DAD system (Thermo Scientific) supplied with an Acclaim 120 C-18 (4.6 × 100 mm) column [21]. For separation, solvent A was water adjusted with acetic acid to pH 2.8, and solvent B was acetonitrile. For flavonoid elution, the gradient was linear to 30% B in 5 min, 45% B in 8 min, and 55% B in 14 min; afterwards the column was washed with 95% B for 3 min and equilibrated for 3 min at 100% A to start the next sample. Total running time was 20 min. Injection volume was 20 µL, and flow rate was 1 mL/min. UV-visible spectra were used to detect flavonoids, and absorbance at 254 nm was used for quantification.

2.11. Water Absorption Index (WAI), Water Solubility Index (WSI) and Expansion Index (EI)

The water absorption index (WAI) and water solubility index (WSI) were assessed before and after the extrusion process [22]. The expansion index (EI) was assessed in seed flour extrudates [22].

2.12. Statistical Analysis

Assays were performed in triplicate, and expressed as means ± standard deviation. Data were submitted to analysis of variance (ANOVA) and means were compared by Tukey test ($p \leq 0.05$).

3. Results and Discussion

3.1. Mesquite Seed Flour Chemical Composition

The chemical composition of mesquite seed flour is shown in Table 1. The main component of mesquite seed flour was nitrogen-free extract (NFE), followed by protein, moisture, crude fiber, fat, and ash. This chemical composition is similar to other seeds of *Prosopis* species, rich in protein and fiber and low in total fat. Previous studies have reported protein contents of 32.3, 62.1 and 30.9 g/100 g in seeds of *P. alba* [9], cotyledons of *P. alba* [14], and seed flour of *P. laevigata* [15], respectively. Previous reported fiber contents in cotyledons of *P. alba* [14], and the seed flour of *P. laevigata* [15] were 9 and 8.3 g/100 g, respectively. Total fat contents of 12.2 and 4 g/100 g have been reported for cotyledons of *P. alba* [14], and seed flour of *P. laevigata* [15], respectively.

Table 1. Chemical composition of mesquite (*Prosopis laevigata*) seed flour.

Component	g/100 g *
Moisture	8.28 ± 0.15
Ash	4.14 ± 0.03
Protein	36.51 ± 0.36
Fat	4.83 ± 0.04
Crude Fiber	7.73 ± 0.46
NFE	38.45 ± 0.66

NFE: nitrogen-free extract. * Values expressed as means ± standard deviation.

Considering legumes seeds from a different genera, the previously reported contents in white lupine of protein, crude fiber, and fat were 34.6, 12.6, and 10 g/100 g, respectively [23]. These values for lentils and common beans were 26.9 and 19.5, 3.1 and 4.4, and 0.8 and 2.4 g/100 g, respectively [23]. Seed flour of *P. laevigata* maintains the healthy nutritional traits, low fat content, and high content of protein and fiber found in legumes, highlighting the potential industrialization of this underutilized legume seed.

3.2. Mesquite Seed Flour Amino Acids Profile

The full amino acid profile of the mesquite seed flour is shown in Table 2. In the present work, four amino acids (Glu, Arg, Asp, and Leu) represented more than 45% of total amino acids, a behavior previously reported for seeds of *P. alba* [14], peas, and common beans [24], but not presented in the soybean [25]. Considering the Food and Agriculture Organization (FAO)-recommended amino acid scoring patterns for humans aged older than 3 years [26], in the present work, Val was the only limiting amino acid in mesquite seed flour. Meanwhile, in seeds of *P. alba*, Lys, Trp, and Thr have been previously reported as limiting amino acids [14]. Trp and sulfur-containing amino acids have been reported as limiting amino acids for peas and common beans, respectively [24]. The seed flour of mesquite is a valuable plant material as a source of good quality protein.

Table 2. Amino acid (AA) profile of mesquite seed flour (mg/g protein).

AA	Seed Flour	* FAO, 2013
Asp	83.4 ± 1.27	
Thr	29.8 ± 0.35	25
Ser	48.1 ± 0.15	
Glu	177.2 ± 2.08	
Pro	62.6 ± 0.95	
Gly	50.6 ± 0.05	
Ala	43.1 ± 0.29	
Val	34.8 ± 0.31	40
Ile	29.2 ± 0.1	30
Leu	69.1 ± 0.45	61
Tyr	22.8 ± 0.61	
Phe	35.6 ± 0.49	
His	24.2 ± 0.3	16
Lys	54.8 ± 0.41	48
Arg	112.2 ± 1.93	
Cis	25.9 ± 0.12	
Met	9.1 ± 0.21	
Trp	6.5 ± 0.22	6.6
Met + Cis	34.9 ± 0.34	23
Phe + Tyr	58.4 ± 1.10	41

* Food and Agriculture Organization (FAO)-recommended amino-acid scoring patterns for humans aged older than 3 years [24]. Values expressed as means ± standard deviation.

3.3. Total Phenolic Compounds, Radical Scavenging Capacity, and Absorbance at 290 nm

Total phenolic compound content, DPPH radical scavenging capacity, and absorbance at 290 nm of seed flour are shown in Table 3. Total phenolic compound content reported here for mesquite seed flour is similar to the previous reported value for *P. laevigata* [15], lower than the value reported for cotyledons of *P. alba* [14], and higher than the respective values reported for lupine, peas, lentils, and common beans [23]. In the present work, the extrusion cooking of mesquite seed flour decreases the content of total phenolic compounds slightly but significantly. DPPH radical scavenging capacity reported here for mesquite seed flour is similar to the previously reported value for *P. laevigata* [15] and higher than the respective values reported for lupine, peas, lentils, and common beans [23]. In the present work, the extrusion cooking of mesquite seed flour increase the DPPH radical scavenging capacity slightly but significantly. The absorbance at 290 nm as an indicator of generation of Maillard reaction products (MRP) was similar in raw and extruded seed flour, suggesting that the extrusion process does not trigger the generation of MRP.

Table 3. Properties of raw and extruded mesquite seed flour.

	Seed Flour *	Extruded Seed Flour *
Total phenolics (mg GAE/g)	6.68 ± 0.05 [a]	6.46 ± 0.06 [b]
DPPH (mg AAE/g)	9.11 ± 0.11 [a]	9.32 ± 0.12 [b]
Abs 290 nm	0.13 ± 0.01 [a]	0.12 ± 0.01 [a]
Apigenin (mg/kg)	41.6 ± 0.51 [a]	39.52 ± 0.47 [b]
WAI	2.53 ± 0.01 [a]	3.47 ± 0.11 [b]
WSI (%)	36.36 ± 0.57 [a]	30.52 ± 0.99 [b]
Expansion index		1

* Values were expressed as means ± standard deviation ($n = 3$). Means accompanied by the same letter in the same line indicate no significant difference between samples ($p < 0.05$). WAI—water absorption index; WSI—water solubility index; GAE—gallic acid equivalent; AAE—ascorbic acid equivalent; DPPH—2-2-diphenyl-1-picrylhydrazyl.

In previous works the generation of Maillard reaction products (assessed as changes in absorbance at 290 nm) during thermal treatment have been associated with increases in the total phenolic compound content and radical scavenging capacity in pods flours of *P. laevigata* [15], flours of carob pods [27], and in synthetic media [20]. The reaction between reducing sugars and amines during thermal treatments produces low molecular weight heterocycles, which can be detected by increases in UV absorbance at 290 nm [20]. These Maillard reaction products have an important free radical scavenging capacity, with reducing activity over the Folin–Ciocalteu reagent in the quantification of total phenolic compounds [15,20]. In some cases, MRP may generate negative effects on human health, resulting in anti-nutritional properties such as the loss of essential amino acids [28]. Flours of mesquite pods have been described as a material very prone to Maillard reaction products generation during baking process [15]. In the presented work the extrusion cooking conditions used for mesquite seed flour processing involves high temperature (150 °C), short time periods (seconds), and low water content (16%); these conditions have been previously suggested for control of MRP generation [28]. Mesquite seed flour is an important source of phenolic compounds with high radical scavenging capacity compared with other legume seeds. Mesquite seed flour extrusion cooking does not affect phenolic compound content or radical scavenging capacity, and does not promote the generation of Maillard reaction products, supporting the use of extrusion technology as an excellent option for mesquite seed flour processing and industrialization.

3.4. Flavonoids

The content of apigenin in raw and extruded mesquite seed flour is shown in Table 3. In the present work, mesquite seed flour was investigated for the presence of myricetin, quercetin, kaempferol, apigenin, daidzein, and genistein. From these flavonoids only the presence of apigenin was confirmed by retention time and UV-VIS spectra. Given the used methodology, the apigenin found in mesquite seed flours corresponds to O-glycosides of apigenin, which were stable to the extrusion cooking process. Previous works reported the presence of C-glycosides of apigenin in pods flours of *P. alba* [11,13,14], and *Prosopis nigra* [29] without quantification. Quercetin, myricetin, and luteolin glycosides have been found in pods flours of *P. alba* [13], Legume seeds have been described as an excellent source of flavonoids; soybean-daidzein and genistein; pea-quercetin, apigenin and kaempferol; common bean-quercetin and kaempferol [21,30,31]. Dietary flavonoids from legumes, including apigenin, have been related with healthy effects on human metabolism through modulation of oxidative stress, hormone function, energetic metabolism, gene expression, and epigenetic process [32–35]. Mesquite seed flour is a source of apigenin, an important active component with healthy implications for humans.

3.5. Water Absorption Index (WAI), Water Solubility Index (WSI) and Expansion Index (EI)

Water absorption index (WAI) and water solubility index (WSI) of raw and extruded mesquite seed flour, together with the expansion index of extruded mesquite seed flour, is shown in Table 3. No previous works were found with respect to *Prosopis* seed flour extrusion. In the present work the extrusion cooking process of mesquite seed flour increases the WAI significantly. Water absorption indicates the amount of water immobilized by the material, as the dispersion by denaturalization of macromolecules such as proteins and starch during extrusion increase the WAI [36], an effect previously described in common bean flours [37]. In the present work the extrusion cooking process of mesquite seed flour decreases the WSI significantly. Water solubility indicates the amount of small molecules solubilized in water, which can be components of the extruded material or can be generated by molecular damage during the extrusion process [36]. Raw mesquite seed flour is a material with water-soluble molecules trapped in the structure formed by the macromolecules denaturalized during extrusion, decreasing the WSI. In the present work the extrusion cooking process of mesquite seed flour produces an extruded material with a poor expansion index, which can be due to the high protein and fiber content in the raw material. High contents of protein and fiber decreased the expansion index of extrudates [38], an effect previously described in corn and common bean-extruded flour blends [39].

Another reported effect of legume seed flour extrusion is the improvement of protein digestibility [40]. The extrusion cooking process of mesquite seed flour modifies the molecular structure of components, improving the nutritional value of the material. Future studies must be conducted in order to develop new extruded products based on mesquite seed flour or in blends with cereals.

4. Conclusions

Mesquite seed flour is a valuable plant food rich in good quality protein and active compounds. The extrusion cooking process of mesquite seed flour is an optional and versatile technology useful in the development of functional foods and industrialization of this underutilized legume.

Author Contributions: Conceptualization, L.D.-B., J.P.H.-U., and C.A.G.-A.; Methodology, R.G.-D., A.T.-J., J.C.-R., and R.P.-C.

Conflicts of Interest: The authors declare no conflict of interest.

References

1. FAO. *Pulses: Nutritious Seeds for a Sustainable Future*; FAO: Rome, Italy, 2016; ISBN 978-92-109463-1.
2. Foyer, C.H.; Lam, H.; Nguyen, H.T.; Siddique, K.H.; Varshney, R.K.; Colmer, T.D.; Cowling, W.; Bramley, H.; Mori, T.A.; Hodgson, J.M.; et al. Neglecting legumes has compromised human health and sustainable food production. *Nat. Plants* **2016**, *2*, 16112. [CrossRef] [PubMed]
3. Singh, B.; Singh, J.P.; Shevkani, K.; Singh, N.; Kaur, A. Bioactive constituents in pulses and their health benefits. *J. Food Sci. Technol.* **2017**, *54*, 858–870. [CrossRef] [PubMed]
4. Iriti, M.; Varoni, E. Pulses, Healthy, and Sustainable Food Sources for Feeding the Planet. *Int. J. Mol. Sci.* **2017**, *18*, 255. [CrossRef] [PubMed]
5. Bhat, R.; Karim, A.A. Exploring the nutritional potential of wild and underutilized legumes. *Compr. Rev. Food Sci. Food Saf.* **2009**, *8*, 305–331. [CrossRef]
6. Morales, P.; Berrios, J.; Varela, J.; Burbano, C.; Cuadrado, C.; Muzquiz, M.; Pedrosa, M. Novel fiber-rich lentil flours as snack-type functional foods: An extrusion cooking effect on bioactive compounds. *Food Funct.* **2015**, *6*, 3135. [CrossRef] [PubMed]
7. El-Hady, E.A.; Habiba, R.A. Effect of soaking and extrusion conditions on antinutrients and protein digestibility of legume seeds. *LWT Food Sci. Technol.* **2003**, *36*, 285–293. [CrossRef]
8. Felker, P.; Takeoka, G.; Dao, L. Pod mesocarp flour of north and south american species of leguminous tree *Prosopis* (Mesquite): Composition and food applications. *Food Rev. Int.* **2013**, *29*, 49–66. [CrossRef]
9. Sciammaro, L.; Ferrero, C.; Puppo, M.C. Chemical and nutritional properties of different fractions of *Prosopis alba* pods and seeds. *Food Meas.* **2015**, *10*, 103–112. [CrossRef]
10. Bigne, F.; Romero, A.; Ferrero, C.; Puppo, M.C.; Guerrero, A. Rheological and microstructural study of wheat doughs partially replaced with Mesquite flour (*Prosopis alba*) and added with transglutaminase. *Food Bioprocess Technol.* **2017**, *10*, 819–830.11. [CrossRef]
11. Schmeda-Hirschmann, G.; Quispe, C.; Soriano, M.P.; Theoduloz, C.; Jiménez-Aspée, F.; Pérez, M.J.; Cuello, A.S.; Isla, M.I. Chilean *Prosopis* Mesocarp Flour: Phenolic Profiling and Antioxidant Activity. *Molecules* **2015**, *20*, 7017–7033. [CrossRef] [PubMed]
12. Huisamen, B.; George, C.; Dietrich, D.; Genade, S. Cardioprotective and anti-hypertensive effects of *Prosopis glandulosa* in rat model of prediabetes. *Cardiovasc. J. Afr.* **2013**, *24*, 10–16. [CrossRef] [PubMed]
13. Young, J.E.; Nguyen, T.; Ly, C.; Jarman, S.; Diep, D.; Pham, C.; Pesek, J.J.; Matyska, M.T.; Takeoka, G.R. LC-MS characterization of Mesquite flour constituents. *LC GC Eur.* **2017**, *30*, 18–21.
14. Cattaneo, F.; Costamagna, M.S.; Zampini, I.C.; Sayago, J.; Alberto, M.R.; Chamorro, V.; Isla, M.I. Flour from *Prosopis alba* cotyledons: A natural source of nutrient and bioactive phytochemicals. *Food Chem.* **2016**, *208*, 89–96. [CrossRef] [PubMed]
15. Díaz-Batalla, L.; Hernández-Uribe, J.-P.; Román-Gutiérrez, A.D.; Cariño-Cortés, R.; Castro-Rosas, J.; Téllez-Jurado, A.; Gómez-Aldapa, C.A. Chemical and nutritional characterization of raw and thermal-treated flours of Mesquite (*Prosopis laevigata*) pods and their residual brans. *CyTA J. Food* **2018**, *16*, 444–451. [CrossRef]
16. AOAC. *Official Methods of Analysis of AOAC International*, 18th ed.; AOAC: Gaithersburg, MD, USA, 2005; ISBN 0-935584-77-3.

17. Li, P.; Zeng, Z.; Wang, D.; Xue, L.; Zhang, R.; Piao, X. Effects of the standardized ileal digestible lysine to metabolizable energy ratio on performance and carcass characteristics of growing-finishing pigs. *J. Anim. Sci. Biotechnol.* **2012**, *3*, 9. [CrossRef] [PubMed]
18. Nielsen, H.; Klein, A.; Hurrell, R. Stability of tryptophan during food processing and storage. *Br. J. Nutr.* **1985**, *53*, 293–300. [CrossRef] [PubMed]
19. Nuutila, A.M.; Kammiovirta, K.; Oksman-Caldentey, K.M. Comparison of methods for the hydrolysis of flavonoids and phenolic acids from onion and spinach for HPLC. *Food Chem.* **2002**, *76*, 519–525. [CrossRef]
20. Yu, X.; Zhao, M.; Hu, J.; Zeng, S.; Bai, X. Correspondence analysis of antioxidant activity and UV-Vis absorbance of Maillard reaction products as related to reactants. *LWT Food Sci. Technol.* **2012**, *46*, 1–9. [CrossRef]
21. Díaz-Batalla, L.; Widholm, J.M.; Fahey, J.C.; Castaño-Tostado, E.; Paredes-López, O. Chemical components with health implications in wild and cultivated Mexican common bean seeds (*Phaseolus vulgaris* L.). *J. Agric. Food Chem.* **2006**, *54*, 2045–2052. [CrossRef] [PubMed]
22. Mesquita, C.; Leonel, M.; Mischan, M.M. Effects of processing on physical properties of extruded snacks with blends of sour cassava starch and flaxseed flour. *Food Sci. Technol. Camp.* **2013**, *33*, 404–410. [CrossRef]
23. Grela, E.R.; Kiczorowska, B.; Samolińska, W.; Matras, J.; Kiczorowski, P.; Rybiński, W.; Hanczakowska, E. Chemical composition of leguminous seeds: Part I—Content of basic nutrients, amino acids, phytochemical compounds, and antioxidant activity. *Eur. Food Res. Technol.* **2017**, *243*, 1385–1395. [CrossRef]
24. Khattab, R.Y.; Arntfield, S.D.; Nyachoti, C.M. Nutritional quality of legume seeds as affected by some physical treatments, Part 1: Protein quality evaluation. *LWT Food Sci. Technol.* **2009**, *42*, 1107–1112. [CrossRef]
25. Yang, H.; Li, X.; Gao, J.; Tong, P.; Yang, A.; Chen, H. Germination-assisted enzymatic hydrolysis can improve the quality of soybean protein. *J. Food Sci.* **2017**, *82*, 1814–1819. [CrossRef] [PubMed]
26. FAO. *Dietary Protein Quality Evaluation in Human Nutrition*; Report of an FAO Expert Consultation; FAO Food and Nutrition Paper 92; FAO: Rome, Italy, 2013; ISBN 978-92-5-107417-6.
27. Sahin, H.; Topuz, A.; Pischetsrieder, M. Effect of roasting process on phenolic, antioxidant and browning properties of carob powder. *Eur. Food Res. Technol.* **2009**, *30*, 155–161. [CrossRef]
28. Lund, M.N.; Ray, C.A. Control of Maillard Reactions in Foods: Strategies and Chemical Mechanisms. *J. Agric. Food Chem.* **2017**, *65*, 4537–4552. [CrossRef] [PubMed]
29. Pérez, M.J.; Zampini, I.C.; Alberto, M.R.; Isla, M.I. *Prosopis nigra* mesocarp fine flour, a source of phytochemicals with potential effect on enzymes linked to metabolic syndrome, oxidative stress, and inflammatory process. *J. Food Sci.* **2018**, *83*, 1454–1462. [CrossRef] [PubMed]
30. Amarowicz, R.; Pegg, R.B. Legumes as a source of natural antioxidants. *Eur. J. Lipid Sci. Technol.* **2008**, *110*, 865–878. [CrossRef]
31. Magalhães, S.; Taveira, M.; Cabrita, A.; Fonseca, A.; Valentão, P.; Andrade, P.B. European marketable grain legume seeds: Further insight into phenolic compounds profiles. *Food Chem.* **2017**, *215*, 177–184. [CrossRef] [PubMed]
32. Sadhukhan, P.; Saha, S.; Sil, P.C. An insight into the prophylactic effects of the leguminosae family plants against oxidative stress-induced pathophysiological conditions. *React. Oxyg. Species* **2018**, *6*, 220–247. [CrossRef]
33. Arangoa, D.; Morohashic, K.; Yilmazc, A.; Kuramochid, K.; Pariharb, A.; Brahimajc, B.; Grotewoldc, E.; Doseff, A. Molecular basis for the action of a dietary flavonoid revealed by the comprehensive identification of apigenin human targets. *Proc. Natl. Acad. Sci. USA* **2013**, *110*, E2153–E2162. [CrossRef] [PubMed]
34. Jung, U.J.; Cho, Y.; Choi, M. Apigenin ameliorates dyslipidemia, hepatic steatosis and insulin resistance by modulating metabolic and transcriptional profiles in the liver of high-fat diet-induced obese mice. *Nutrients* **2016**, *8*, 305. [CrossRef] [PubMed]
35. Kanwal, R.; Datt, M.; Liu, X.; Gupta, S. Dietary flavones as dual Inhibitors of DNA methyltransferases and histone methyltransferases. *PLoS ONE* **2016**, *11*, e162956. [CrossRef]
36. Oikonomou, N.A.; Krokida, M.K. Literature data compilation of WAI and WSI of extrudate foods products. *Int. J. Food Prop.* **2011**, *14*, 199–240. [CrossRef]
37. Natabirwa, H.; Muyonga, J.; Nakimbugwea, D.; Lungahoc, M. Physico-chemical properties and extrusion behaviour of selected common bean varieties. *J. Sci. Food Agric.* **2017**, *98*, 1492–1501. [CrossRef] [PubMed]

38. Alam, M.S.; Kaur, J.; Khaira, H.; Gupta, K. Extrusion and extruded products: Changes in quality attributes as affected by extrusion process parameters: A review. *Crit. Rev. Food Sci. Nutr.* **2016**, *56*, 445–473. [CrossRef] [PubMed]
39. Lazou, A.E.; Michailidis, P.A.; Thymi, S.; Krokida, M.K.; Bisharat, G.I. Structural properties of corn-legume based extrudates as a function of processing conditions and raw material characteristics. *Int. J. Food Prop.* **2007**, *10*, 721–738. [CrossRef]
40. Patil, S.S.; Brennan, M.A.; Mason, S.L.; Brennan, C.S. The effects of fortification of legumes and extrusion on the protein digestibility of wheat based snack. *Foods* **2016**, *5*, 26. [CrossRef] [PubMed]

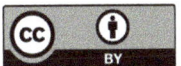

© 2018 by the authors. Licensee MDPI, Basel, Switzerland. This article is an open access article distributed under the terms and conditions of the Creative Commons Attribution (CC BY) license (http://creativecommons.org/licenses/by/4.0/).

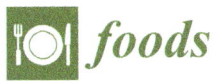

Article

Effect of Traditional Household Processes on Iron, Zinc and Copper Bioaccessibility in Black Bean (*Phaseolus vulgaris* L.)

Sabrina Feitosa [1,2,*], **Ralf Greiner** [1], **Ann-Katrin Meinhardt** [1], **Alexandra Müller** [1], **Deusdélia T. Almeida** [2] **and Clemens Posten** [3]

1. Department of Food Technology and Bioprocess Engineering, Max Rubner Institut, Federal Research Institute of Nutrition and Food, Haid-und-Neu-Str. 9, D-76131 Karlsruhe, Germany; ralf.greiner@mri.bund.de (R.G.); ann-katrin.meinhardt@mri.bund.de (A.-K.M.); alexandra.mueller@mri.bund.de (A.M.)
2. School of Nutrition, Federal University of Bahia, Av. Araújo Pinho 32, Salvador 40110-150, Brazil; deliata@uol.com.br
3. Institute of Life Science Engineering, Bioprocess Engineering, University of Karlsruhe, Fritz-Haber-Weg 2, 76131 Karlsruhe, Germany; clemens.posten@kit.edu
* Correspondence: sabrinafeitosa0@gmail.com; Tel.: +49-(0)721-6625-328

Received: 29 June 2018; Accepted: 30 July 2018; Published: 31 July 2018

Abstract: Micronutrient deficiencies are a major public health problem. Beans are an important plant-based source of iron, zinc and copper, but their absorption is reduced in the presence of anti-nutrients such as phytates, polyphenols and tannins. Soaking and discarding the soaking water before cooking is unanimously recommended, but this can result in mineral loss. Data on the consequences for mineral bioaccessibility is still limited. This study aimed to evaluate iron, zinc and copper bioaccessibility in black beans cooked (regular pan, pressure cooker) with and without the soaking water. For that, three batches of black beans were investigated in triplicate, each split in nine parts (raw grains and four different household processes in duplicate) and analyzed by applying the quarter technique, resulting in a grand total of 164 samples. Minerals were quantified by ICP-MS (inductively coupled plasma mass spectrometry), *myo*-inositol phosphates (InsP$_5$, InsP$_6$) by HPLC (high-performance liquid chromatography) ion-pair chromatography, total polyphenols using Folin-Denis reagent and condensed tannins using Vanillin assay. Mineral bioaccessibility was determined by in vitro digestion and dialysis. All treatments resulted in a statistically significant reduction of total polyphenols (30%) and condensed tannins (20%). Only when discarding the soaking water a loss of iron (6%) and copper (30%) was observed, and InsP$_6$ was slightly decreased (7%) in one treatment. The bioaccessibility of iron and zinc were low (about 0.2% iron and 35% zinc), but copper presented high bioaccessibility (about 70%). Cooking beans under pressure without discarding the soaking water resulted in the highest bioaccessibility levels among all household procedures. Discarding the soaking water before cooking did not improve the nutritional quality of the beans.

Keywords: beans; iron; zinc and copper bioaccessibility; *myo*-inositol phosphates; anti-nutrients; polyphenols; household processing

1. Introduction

Deficiencies of micronutrients are a major public health problem, in which iron and zinc malnutrition affects more than half of the population worldwide [1,2]. Iron-deficiency anemia reaches more than 30% of the world's population, approximately 20% in European Union and up to 40% in developing countries [1,3]. It contributes to 20% of maternal deaths besides being related to low adult productivity at work [3,4]. Outcomes of zinc deficiency are depressed growth, immune dysfunction, lower respiratory tract infections, diarrhea, altered cognition and other clinical conditions [4,5]. Copper deficiency may also lead to anemia, but features of human copper deficiency mechanisms are still unknown [6], while most copper research is focused on soil, fruits and nuts e.g., [7,8].

The major reason for iron deficiency is a poor availability of iron from the diet. Mineral deficiencies are not only caused by low dietary intake. Many other factors affect the absorption such as the total content of the minerals and anti-nutrients, the processing applied and mineral interactions [9,10]. The interactions concerning iron, zinc and copper appear to be especially important, and the bioaccessibility is influenced differently depending on the mineral [11,12]. Dietary and human factors, such as inflammation and disease, have been found to be the major factors influencing the bioavailability of micronutrients. Dietary factors are related to food matrix structure and composition, being mostly influenced by the interaction with other dietary compounds, such as fibers, lipids, proteins and anti-nutrients during digestion and absorption. It is also important to consider not only the total content of iron, zinc and copper in crops, but also the tissue localization (cotyledon and endosperm) and specification (chelates and protein particles) [11,13]. Iron exists in two different forms in food: hemic iron in animal products and non-hemic iron in plant foods which is generally poorly absorbed. Iron is stored in plants and animals as the protein ferritin, and about 80% of the iron in beans is present in the form of non-ferritin-bound iron which is possibly bound to *myo*-inositol phosphates [11,14]. Condensed tannins are able to form tannin-protein complexes that can chelate iron and calcium. Animal studies have demonstrated that in the presence of phytate, calcium can impair zinc absorption, probably by co-precipitation with phytate and zinc. Furthermore, digestibility and hence absorption of micronutrients such as iron and zinc can be improved upon heat processing, which results in softening of the food matrix, with release of protein-bound iron and zinc, thus facilitating its absorption. Studies in human subjects have shown that zinc may stimulate iron absorption, and calcium can inhibit iron absorption by inhibiting iron transport. Copper is essential for iron transport between tissues in which iron and copper homeostases are linked by the inability to export iron to the systemic circulation in the absence of copper. On the mechanistic level, neither zinc nor calcium seem to be as crucial for iron absorption as copper, but there are only few studies about copper deficiency and sufficient copper levels in the diet [6,11,12].

Beans are highly nutritious and the most consumed leguminous grain worldwide, which are an important plant-based source of iron, zinc and copper [15–17]. They are part of many traditional diets, playing a major role in vegetarian diets in all countries, besides being consumed in different dishes together with other food products [9,15,17,18]. Therefore, mineral bioavailability may also be influenced by interference with other food constituents [9,10]. Common beans are a staple food in Latin America and Eastern Africa [19,20] and Brazil is the most important consumer of beans in the world, with up to 19 kg/year per capita consumption, 80% of which is common bean and black bean is the second most consumed [17,21]. Approximately, a portion per meal of cooked beans (100 g) [15,17] contains 6.52–10.00 mg iron, 0.93–1.21 mg copper and 3.18–3.60 mg zinc, which equals the daily requirements for healthy adults for iron and copper and half of that of zinc (8 mg/day, 0.9 mg/day and 8–11 mg/day, respectively) [22]. Therefore, a regular intake of beans could contribute to minimize deficiencies of micronutrients [15,17]. The nutritional quality of beans, however, is usually reduced by the presence of anti-nutrients, such as phytates, polyphenols and tannins [9,20]. Those compounds bind to minerals such as iron, zinc, copper, calcium and magnesium, thus reducing bioavailability due to the formation of extremely insoluble salts or very poorly dissociated chelates.

Phytates (InsP$_6$), have especially been reported to affect iron and zinc absorption negatively even at low concentrations [9,23–25]. Condensed tannins are able to form tannin-protein complexes, which can chelate iron and calcium [9,26,27]. A reduction of mineral bioavailability was observed when condensed tannins concentration was higher than 10% of the total dry weight of the samples or ranging from 2.5 to 4.7 mg eq. CE g^{-1} [27,28]. With regard to polyphenolic compounds, it has been reported that they reduce bioavailability of some minerals. Although there is no consensus on the quantity needed to decrease iron absorption in beans, a reduction in iron bioavailability was observed above 50 mg of polyphenols [27,29]. Furthermore, the polyphenols in legumes have been extensively correlated with health benefits in humans due to their potent anti-oxidant activities [30,31]. In common beans, those bioactive compounds mostly comprise phenolic acids and condensed tannins which are found in the cotyledons, and exhibit anti-diabetic, anti-obesity, anti-inflammatory, anti-mutagenic and anti-carcinogenic effects [30–32].

In a recent study [33], polyphenols of black beans were individually examined for their effect on iron uptake by Caco-2 cells. Half of the polyphenols studied were shown to inhibit iron absorption, but the other half were found to clearly promote iron absorption. So far, many studies [23,24,27,34] reported the link between a reduction of the total content of anti-nutrients in food grains with a higher availability of iron and zinc. Food processing and food preparation techniques like soaking, germination, hydrothermal treatment and fermentation can reduce the content of anti-nutrients [9,25,34]. Soaking and discarding the soaking water before cooking beans has been unanimously recommended due to a higher reduction of the anti-nutrients. An average reduction of 20% to 30% of condensed tannins and total polyphenols can be obtained in legumes by applying household processes [27,34,35]. The effect on mineral bioavailability was assessed in those studies mainly by molar ratios and statistical correlations between the content of anti-nutrients and the mineral content [27,34,35]. In general, digestibility and not bioavailability assays were applied in those studies. Bioavailability and bioaccessibility are often used indistinctly [36].

Only direct feeding trials can fully determine biological efficacy and mineral interactions, but they are long-lasting, cost intensive, and nonetheless the results need to be extrapolated to the human organism. A simple method to estimate the effect of for example food processing on mineral bioavailability is the use of bioaccessibility assays [19,24]. Although there is a substantial amount of information about binding of iron and zinc, and anti-nutrients reduction by food processing, data on the consequences for mineral absorption are still limited. Discarding the soaking water before cooking beans can result in loss of minerals and anti-oxidants and thus the nutritional quality of cooked beans is not necessarily improved. Thus, this study aimed to evaluate iron, zinc and copper bioaccessibility in black beans cooked with and without the soaking water using traditional household processes in order to expand knowledge about the nutritional value of this basic and accessible food and the options to use beans in combating micronutrients deficiencies.

2. Materials and Methods

All glassware used in sample preparation and analyses was washed in distilled water and for mineral analysis also immersed in a 5% nitric acid solution for more than 1 h and rinsed with ultrapure water (Milli-Q, Millipore, Merck KGaA, Darmstadt, Germany). The following describes in details the methods for analyzing three batches of black beans in triplicate, each split in nine parts (raw grains and four different household processes in duplicate), which were studied by applying the quarter technique, resulting in a total of 164 samples.

2.1. Samples

Three different batches of common beans (*Phaseolus vulgaris* L., black bean variety) from three randomly selected markets in Rio de Janeiro, Brazil, were used in this study. All batches were from commercial cultivation, geographic origin in the region of São Paulo, $-23°10'45''$ S, $45°53'12''$ W, and harvested in June–July of 2015. The procedures applied during growth of the crop were not available. Moreover, the influence of the crop season on the black beans of this study is negligible [37]. The black bean samples were sent to Germany (Max Rubner-Institut, Karlsruhe, Germany), where the study (including the household processing) was performed in a period of one year, in a controlled environment to mitigate the influence of seasons to the experiment. The samples were stored at 4 °C with an extra vacuum-packaging. The raw grains were cleaned before use. All dirt was removed manually and then the beans were washed with deionized water. After that, the beans were cooked. For analyses the samples were freeze-dried (developed at the Max Rubner-Institut, Karlsruhe, Germany, operating with an air temperature of $-30\,°C$ and air velocity of 6 ms^{-1}) and finely ground in a stainless steel analytical grinder (A10 Yellow Line, IKA-Werke GmbH & Co. KG, Staufen, Germany). Thereafter, a quarter technique was applied to the raw grains and the cooked beans together with the broth in order to obtain two final fractions properly homogenized. Each analytical determination was carried out in triplicate for each fraction of cooked and raw samples.

2.2. Household Treatments

In order to simulate traditional household processes for cooking beans, an overnight soaking (12 h) at room temperature was performed, followed by two cooking methods (boiling and pressure cooking) in tap water. Three different batches of black beans were used. A proportion of 100 g of the black beans and 400 mL of water were used for soaking. The following cooking strategies were performed: (1) with the soaking water in a pressure cooker; (2) without the soaking water in a pressure cooker; (3) with the soaking water in a regular pan; and (4) without the soaking water in a regular pan. The regular pan had a capacity of 3 L and the beans were cooked for 35 min. 200 mL of tap water were added during cooking to replenish the loss of evaporated water. The pressure cooker had a capacity of 3 L and the beans were cooked for 5 min. No water was added during the cooking process. The cooking times were chosen according to the results of a test cooking simulation. Before cooking the black beans, either tap water was added to the soaking water to give a final volume of 600 mL or the soaking water was discarded and replaced by tap water to give a final volume of 600 mL. All treatments were performed in duplicate for each batch of black beans. The same cooking methods were also performed without bean samples to quantify the concentrations of the minerals in the water before and after the cooking process.

2.3. Myo-Inositol Phosphates

Quantification of *myo*-inositol phosphates was performed by extracting 1 g of a freeze-dried sample with 20 mL of 2.4% HCl for 3 h with constant shaking at room temperature. The resulting suspensions were centrifuged (30 min, 15,000 rpm). The supernatant was collected and used for *myo*-inositol phosphate quantification [38]; 2 mL of the supernatant were diluted with ultrapure water to give a final volume of 60 mL. The entire solution was applied to a column (0.7 × 15 cm) containing 0.5 g of AG 1–X4 100–200-mesh resin (Bio-Rad Laboratories GmbH, München, Germany). The column was washed with 25 mL of ultrapure water and 25 mL of 25 mM HCl. Then *myo*-inositol phosphates were eluted with 25 mL of 2 M HCl. The eluates obtained were concentrated in a vacuum evaporator (Rotavapor RE-120, BÜCHI Labortechnik AG, Flawil, Switzerland) (at 40 °C) and dissolved in 1 mL of ultrapure water. Then 20 µL of the samples were chromatographed on Ultrasep ES 100 RP18 (2 × 250 mm). The column was run at 40 °C and 0.2 mL min^{-1} of an eluent consisting of formic acid/methanol/water/tetrabutylammonium hydroxide (44:56:5:1.5 v/v), pH 4.25. A mixture of the individual *myo*-inositol phosphate esters (InsP$_3$–InsP$_6$) was used as a standard [39]. The retention times of InsP$_5$ and InsP$_6$ were 15 min and 23 min, respectively.

2.4. Total Polyphenols

Total phenols were extracted with water. An internal standard curve was prepared by adding 10 mL of 0–0.01% tannic acid to the flasks. The flasks were heated for 30 min at 70 °C with constant shaking. Clear supernatants were collected after centrifugation at 2500 g for 15 min followed by filtration. Polyphenols were determined using the Folin–Denis reagent [40].

2.5. Condensed Tannins

Condensed tannins were extracted with HCl:methanol (1:100 v/v) for 2 h with mechanical shaking (Universal shaker SM, Carl Roth GmbH + Co. KG, Karlsruhe, Germany) at 25 °C and centrifuged

(Sorvall LYNX 6000, Thermo Scientific, Langenselbold, Germany) at 5000 g at 15 °C for 15 min. Aliquots were immediately analyzed for tannins using the 0.5% vanillin assay [41].

2.6. Minerals

Iron (Fe), zinc (Zn), copper (Cu) and calcium (Ca) concentrations were measured. Therefore, 150 mg of each ground sample was microwave-digested in a MWS–1 (Berghof Products + Instruments GmbH, Eningen, Germany) with 3 mL of concentrated HNO_3 (65% v/v) and 0.75 mL of H_2O_2 (30% v/v). Heating was performed in four successive steps: linear temperature increased up to 150 °C in 5 min (80 W); 5 min at 150 °C (70 W); linear temperature increased up to 180 °C in 40 min (80 W); 10 min at 180 °C (80 W). All samples were analyzed in triplicate and a set of digestion blanks were prepared with each sample batch. The data was expressed as mean ± standard deviation on dry matter (DM) basis.

Element analysis was performed by inductively coupled plasma mass spectrometry (ICP-MS), iCAP Q (Thermo Scientific, Waltham, MA, USA). The ICP-MS operating conditions and measurement parameters are given in Table 1. Standard addition was used for calibration. The limit of quantification (LOQ) was calculated based on the measured values of the blanks (n = 152), where LOQ = mean + 10× standard deviation. The extreme studentized deviate test was used to remove outliers from the data set. Fresh kidney beans NCS ZC73019 (GSB–12) was used as reference material (n = 84) to determine precision and accuracy of the method (Table 2). The relative standard deviations were less than 3% for all investigated elements, and at a 95% confidence level showed that there was no significant difference between the means of the certified and determined values for the analytes under investigation.

Table 1. ICP-MS operating conditions and measurement parameters.

Parameter	Value
Radiofrequency power	1550 W
Argon flow rates	
Cooling	13.8 L min^{-1}
Auxiliary	0.65 L min^{-1}
Nebulizer	1.05 L min^{-1}
Sample cone	Ni
Skimmer cone	Ni
Analyte	43Ca, 56Fe, 65Cu, 66Zn
Internal standard	103Rh (Fe, Cu, Zn), 45Sc (Ca, Fe), 89Y (Fe, Cu), 72Ge (Ca, Zn), 115In (Cu, Zn)
Aquisition/scanning mode	STD (Ca), KED (Fe, Cu, Zn)
Sweeps per reading	100
Dwell time	10 ms (Ca, Cu, Zn); 40 ms (Fe)
No. of runs	5
Replicate time	21 s
Sample uptake rate	0.2 mL min^{-1}
Wash time between samples (2% HNO_3)	30 s
Sample delay	50 s
Stabilization time	5 s

ICP-MS: Inductively Coupled Plasma Mass Spectrometry.

Table 2. ICP-MS precision and accuracy of the method.

Element	LOQ (µg kg^{-1})	Reference Material Measured Value (mg kg^{-1})	Reference Material Certificate Value (mg kg^{-1})
Ca	29.8	0.66 ± 0.06	0.67 ± 0.04
Fe	1.8	306 ± 29	330 ± 20
Cu	7.2	8.4 ± 1.5	8.7 ± 0.5
Zn	6.6	34 ± 4	32 ± 2

LOQ: limit of quantification.

2.7. Iron, Zinc and Copper Bioaccessibility

In order to be able to quantify bioaccessibility in cooked black bean samples, a simplified *in vitro* gastrointestinal digestion assay was carried out. Iron, zinc and copper bioaccessibilities were determined based on *in vitro* digestion and dialysis method described by [42] with modifications.

For gastric digestion, 10 g of ground sample were suspended in 60 mL of 20 mM glycine-HCl buffer, pH 2.0. After, adjusting pH to 2.0 by with 2 M HCl, 1.3 mL of pepsin (porcine, Fluka Analytical, Sigma-Aldrich Chemie GmbH, Steinheim, Germany) solution (1.6 g pepsin in 10 mL 20 mM glycine-HCl buffer, pH 2.0) were added. The suspension was incubated at 37 °C for 2 h under agitation. To simulate intestinal digestion, the pH of the gastric digestion was adjusted to 7.2 with 1 M $NaHCO_3$. 13 mL of a pancreatin (porcine, P1750, Sigma-Aldrich Chemie GmbH, Steinheim, Germany) solution (0.4 g pancreatin in 100 mL of ultrapure water) were added and a dialysis bag (cut of 10,000 Da; Carl Roth GmbH + Co. KG, Karlsruhe, Germany, containing 2 mL of ultrapure water) was placed in the digestion system. The system was incubated at 37 °C for 2 h, under agitation. Thereafter, the dialysis bag was removed and iron, zinc and copper in the dialysate were analyzed by ICP-MS. Bioaccessibility (%) was calculated as $100 \times Y/Z$ whereby Y represents the dialyzable amount of the mineral per 100 g DM of cooked beans and Z the total of the same mineral per 100 g DM of the cooked beans.

2.8. Statistical Analysis

All the analyses were conducted in triplicate and expressed as mean ± standard deviation of three separate determinations. The results were evaluated for normality by the Shapiro–Wilk test. The data generated was subjected to one-way analysis of variance (ANOVA) using the software Sigma Plot version 13.0. A Tukey's paired comparison test was used to determine statistically significant differences ($p < 0.05$) among the batches and in between raw and treated samples mean values, at a 95% confidence level.

3. Results and Discussion

3.1. Mineral Contents of Raw and Cooked Beans

The mean iron, zinc, copper and calcium contents of the three black bean batches are presented in Figure 1. All batches were not significantly different ($p > 0.05$) among each other.

Black beans were confirmed to be a good source of iron, zinc and copper. Approximately a portion per meal of cooked black beans (100 g) contains an average of 6.5 mg iron, 4 mg zinc and 1 mg copper. Those contents are in good agreement with data published by the Food and Agriculture Organization of the United Nations database [15] for common beans of the same origin. Thus, 100 g of black bean meets the daily requirement for copper (0.9 mg/day), and partially that for iron (8 mg/day) and zinc (8–11 mg/day) [22].

Discarding the soaking water before cooking the beans resulted in a lower content ($p < 0.001$) of iron (6%) and copper (30%) compared to the raw beans (Figure 1A,B). According to Raes et al. [13], the differences in leaching of micronutrients can be attributed to the fact that these minerals are bound by different food constituents with different binding strength. Furthermore, their location within the food matrix might be different. Zinc and calcium contents was found to be increased irrespective of the household procedure applied ($p < 0.001$). The highest contents (Zn: 132–150%, Ca: 191%) were found in black beans cooked in a regular pan (Figure 1C,D).

The concentrations of the minerals in the water before and after the cooking process were measured and hence either present in the tap water or released from the pressure cooker or pan. Iron and copper concentrations of the tap water before and after cooking were below the LOQ (mg 100 g^{-1}): Fe (0.14), Cu (0.56). Zinc mean concentrations were determined to be below the LOQ (0.51 mg 100 mL^{-1}) in the tap water. In the boiled water samples, it ranged from 0.75 ± 0.06 mg (pressure cooker) to 1.92 ± 0.32 mg (regular pan). Therefore, the increase in the Zn contents was found to be due to a leaching of zinc ions from the pan surface. A smaller increase ($p < 0.05$) in Zn content (123–125%) was also observed during pressure cooking (Figure 1C). Katzenberg et al. [43], also reported higher zinc concentrations in beef as an effect of the cooking method and Quintaes et al. [44], have shown the migration of metal ions from cookware into foods.

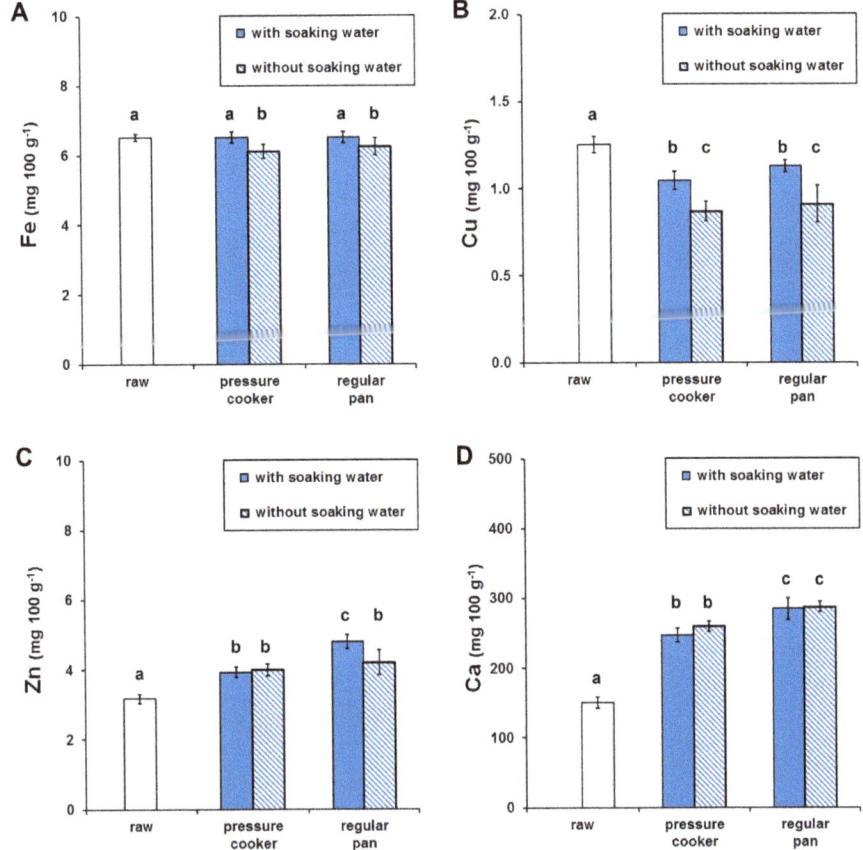

Figure 1. Black bean contents of iron (**A**), copper (**B**), zinc (**C**) and calcium (**D**). Data expressed as mean ± standard deviation (dry matter). Values marked by different letters are significantly different ($p < 0.05$).

The mean Ca concentration in the tap water was determined to be 16.83 ± 1.38 mg 100 mL^{-1}. Thus, the theoretical amount of calcium added was 100.98 mg 100 g^{-1} for pressure cooking and 134.64 mg 100 g^{-1} in the regular pan. The observed increases in calcium were found to be 97.00 ± 1.57 mg 100 g^{-1} (with soaking water) and 109.27 ± 0.61 mg 100 g^{-1} (without soaking water) for pressure cooking, and 134.66 ± 7.23 mg 100 g^{-1} (with soaking water) and 136.95 ± 0.80 mg 100 g^{-1} (without soaking water) using the regular pan (Figure 1D). Therefore, the increase in Ca contents was due to the addition of tap water during cooking.

3.2. Anti-Nutrients

The mean contents of InsP$_6$, InsP$_5$, total polyphenols and condensed tannins are presented in Figure 2. All traditional household processes applied resulted in a statistically significant reduction in total polyphenols (about 30%) and condensed tannins (about 20%) compared to raw black bean (Figure 2C,D). Discarding the soaking water before cooking the beans resulted in a greater reduction of polyphenols and tannins, which is in good accordance with the majority of studies [27,34]. Since polyphenols of legumes have been extensively correlated with health benefits in humans due to their potent anti-oxidant activities [30–32], their reduction during processing does not necessarily improve the nutritional quality of beans. With regard to *myo*-inositol phosphates, only with beans cooked without the soaking water in a pressure cooker a slightly decrease (7%) in $InsP_6$ content was observed. $InsP_5$ contents, however, increased with all cooking procedures applied. Furthermore, no statistical difference was observed among the three batches of the black bean samples regarding the contents of anti-nutrients.

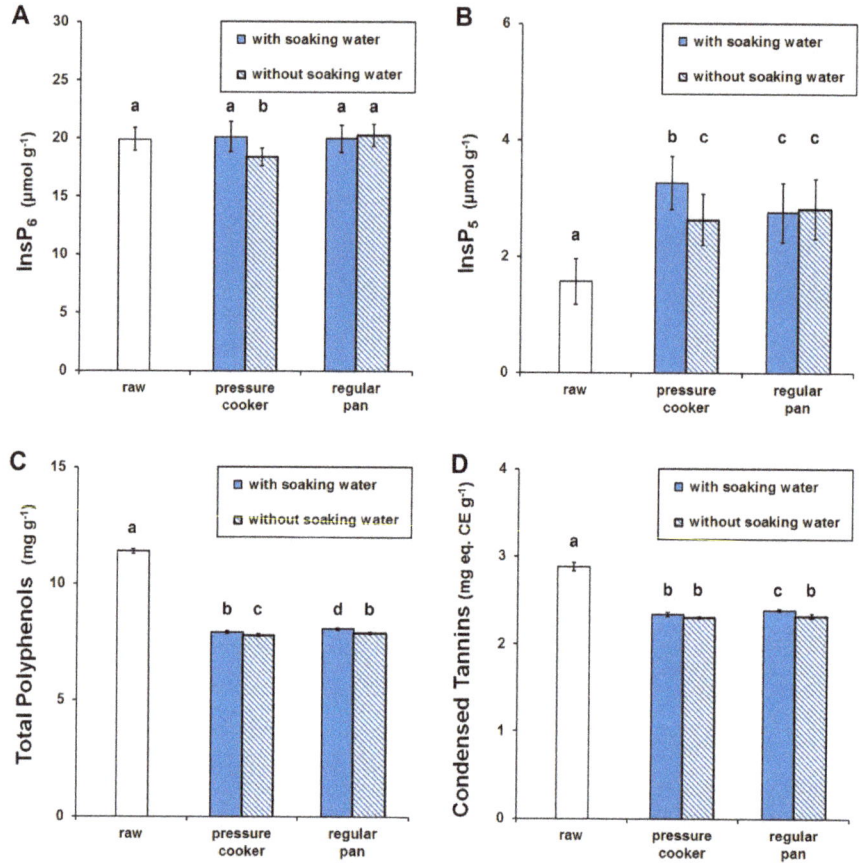

Figure 2. Black bean anti-nutrients content of $InsP_6$ (**A**), $InsP_5$ (**B**), total polyphenols (**C**) and condensed tannins (**D**). Data expressed as mean ± standard deviation (dry matter). Values marked by different letters are significantly different ($p < 0.05$).

3.3. Bioaccessibility of Iron, Zinc and Copper

The mean levels (%) of iron, zinc and copper bioaccessibility in cooked black beans are shown in Table 3. The determination of the micronutrient bioaccessibility makes it possible to estimate the percentage of absorption of those minerals with a simple and affordable assay compared to bioavailability assessment. Beans are highly nutritious legumes that have been reported as one of the best plant-based sources of bioaccessible iron and zinc [18–20]. In this study however, iron bioaccessibility levels were found to be low with all household processes (Table 3). On the other hand, copper showed high bioaccessibility, followed by zinc (Table 3).

Table 3. Bioaccessibility levels (%) of iron, zinc and copper in black bean cooked with traditional household processes.

Household Processes	Iron (%)	Zinc (%)	Copper (%)
Regular pan with soaking water	0.18 [a]	33.94 [a]	71.53 [a]
Pressure cooker with soaking water	0.33 [b]	44.66 [b]	73.35 [a]
Regular pan without soaking water	0.17 [a]	31.55 [a]	66.42 [b]
Pressure cooker without soaking water	0.22 [a]	35.04 [a]	68.16 [b]

In each column, values marked by different letters are a significantly different ($p < 0.05$).

Recent reviews [27,34] reported a link between iron and zinc availability from common beans and cooking soaked beans without the soaking water. This was reported to be due to the reduction of the content in anti-nutrients during food processing [9]. In this present study, however, black bean cooked with the soaking water in a pressure cooker resulted in the highest bioaccessibility for all three minerals in spite of higher total anti-nutrients reduction in beans cooked without the soaking water. According to Hoppler et al. [14], 70–85% of the iron in beans is present in the form of non-ferritin-bound iron and it is possibly bound to *myo*-inositol phosphates. Phytate is abundant in legumes, cereals and nuts, being considered to be the most powerful anti-nutrient due to their high binding capacity for metals and also their ability to form large insoluble aggregates [23,25].

Discarding the soaking water was shown to have a negative effect on the bioaccessibility of all three minerals in regular pan. Assessing mineral bioavailability in those studies mainly by molar ratios and statistical correlations between the content of anti-nutrients and the mineral content might be responsible for the observed differences in the obtained results [27,34,35]. In addition, details on the cooking methods applied were not reported. Pereira et al. [19], studied the effect of household cooking methods on the bioaccessibility of iron and zinc in different beans cultivars. Iron bioaccessibility of beans cooked with the soaking water in a pressure cooker were higher (6.46–40.68%) compared to beans cooked in a regular pan (2.42–8.92%). In the present study, the same tendency was observed. Even if lower Fe bioaccessibilities were found in this study, Zn bioaccessibilities were observed to be always higher than Fe bioaccessibilities. Bioaccessibility studies are a useful method to estimate the general trend of a household procedure on mineral bioavailability, but the absolute data obtained in those studies do not represent the situation in a human digestive tract. Neither active mineral uptake nor the interaction of minerals with respect to binding to food constituents or interaction with mineral transporters in the small intestine can be considered through bioaccessibility studies. The interactions concerning iron, zinc and copper appear to be of utmost importance in respect to their bioavailability [11,12]. Since micronutrient uptake has been successfully studied by Caco-2 cells models due to their exclusive ability to model human absorption characteristics [45–47], the data obtained in this study should be confirmed using a Caco-2 cell model.

4. Conclusions

Black beans were confirmed to be a good source of iron, zinc and copper with a high bioaccessibility of copper (about 70%) from cooked beans. The bioaccessibility of iron and zinc, however, were found to be low (about 0.2% for iron and 35% for zinc). Cooking beans under pressure without discarding the soaking water resulted in the highest bioaccessibility levels among all household procedures applied. Although a reduction in anti-nutrients' content was observed, the *myo*-inositol phosphate content did not change significantly. In addition, discarding the soaking water before cooking the beans did not improve their nutritional quality. This procedure resulted in a loss of iron, copper and bioactive compounds.

Data on the consequences for iron, zinc and copper absorption are still limited. Thus, improving knowledge about the influence of traditional household processes on the nutritional value of this basic and accessible food is important. Further work is necessary to increase especially iron availability in home-cooked beans. Since phytate is the constituent with the highest impact on mineral bioavailability in common beans, applying the most efficient household procedures combined with phytase application might be a promising approach.

Author Contributions: Conceptualization, Project Administration and Investigation, Funding Acquisition, Formal Analysis, Writing—Original Draft Preparation & Visualization, S.F.; Writing—Review and Editing, R.G. and D.T.A.; Methodology, Data Curation, Review and Editing, A.-K.M., A.M., R.G. and S.F. Supervision, R.G. and C.P.

Funding: This research was funded by Conselho Nacional de Desenvolvimento Científico e Tecnológico (CNPq) grant number 234524/2014-6.

Acknowledgments: All technical support and materials used for experiments of the Max Rubner-Instiut and the Department of Food Technology and Bioprocess Engineering.

Conflicts of Interest: The authors declare no conflict of interest and the funders had no role in the design of the study, in the collection, analyses, or interpretation of data; in the writing of the manuscript, and in the decision to publish the results.

Limitations: Although this study was carefully conducted and has reached its aim, there was an unavoidable limitation. The specified information regarding what procedures were applied during growth of the crop is not available for the commercial cultivation of black beans used in this research. In addition, to mitigate the influence of seasons when the study was conducted, the experiments were performed entirely in a controlled environment.

References

1. World Health Organization (WHO). Nutrition Topics. Micronutrient Deficiencies. Available online: http://www.who.int/nutrition/topics/micronutrients/en/ (accessed on 23 May 2018).
2. World Health Organization (WHO). The World Health Report 2002: Reducing Risks, Promoting Healthy Life. Available online: http://www.who.int/whr/2002/en/whr02_en.pdf (accessed on 23 May 2018).
3. World Health Organization (WHO). World Health Statistics. Available online: www.who.int/whosis/whostat/2011/en/ (accessed on 23 May 2018).
4. World Health Organization (WHO). Global Health Risks, Part 2, Results. Available online: http://www.who.int/healthinfo/global_burden_disease/GlobalHealthRisks_report_part2.pdf (accessed on 30 May 2018).
5. Hambidge, K.M. Mild zinc deficiency in human subjects. In *Zinc in Human Biology*; Mills, C.F., Ed.; Springer: New York, NY, USA, 1989; pp. 281–296.
6. Lazarchick, J. Update on anemia and neutropenia in copper deficiency. *Curr. Opin. Hematol.* **2012**, *19*, 58–60. [CrossRef] [PubMed]
7. Lamb, D.T.; Ming, H.; Megharaj, M.; Naidu, R. Heavy metal (Cu, Zn, Cd and Pb) partitioning and bioaccessibility in uncontaminated and long-term contaminated soils. *J. Hazard Mater.* **2009**, *171*, 1150–1158. [CrossRef]
8. Lima, A.C.S.; Soares, D.J.; Silva, L.M.R.; Figueiredo, R.W.; Sousa, P.H.M.; Menezes, E.A. In Vitro bioaccessibility of copper, iron, zinc and antioxidant compounds of whole cashew apple juice and cashew apple fibre (*Anacardium occidentale* L.) following simulated gastro-intestinal digestion. *Food Chem.* **2014**, *161*, 142–147. [CrossRef] [PubMed]
9. Sandberg, A.S. Bioavailability of minerals in legumes. *Br. J. Nutr.* **2002**, *88*, 281–285. [CrossRef]
10. Cozzolino, S.M.F. Biodisponibilidade de minerais. *Rev. Nutr.* **1997**, *88*, 87–98. [CrossRef]
11. Scheers, N. Regulatory effects of Cu, Zn, and Ca on Fe absorption: The intricate play between nutrient transporters. *Nutrients* **2013**, *5*, 957–970. [CrossRef] [PubMed]
12. Olivares, M.; Pizarro, F.; Ruz, M.; De Romaña, D.L. Acute inhibition of iron bioavailability by zinc: Studies in humans. *Biometals* **2012**, *25*, 657–664. [CrossRef]
13. Raes, K.; Knockaert, D.; Struijs, K.; Van Camp, J. Role of processing on bioaccessibility of minerals: Influence of localization of minerals and anti-nutritional factors in the plant. *Trends Food Sci. Technol.* **2014**, *37*, 32–41. [CrossRef]
14. Hoppler, M.; Zeder, C.; Walczyk, T. Quantification of ferritin-bound iron in plant samples by isotope tagging and species-specific isotope dilution mass spectrometry. *Anal. Chem.* **2009**, *81*, 7368–7372. [CrossRef] [PubMed]
15. Food and Agriculture Organization of the United Nations (FAO). FAO/INFOODS Global Food Composition Database for Pulses Version 1.0-uPulses 1.0. Available online: http://www.fao.org/infoods/infoods/tables-and-databases/faoinfoods-databases/en/ (accessed on 30 April 2018).

16. Akibode, S.; Maredia, M.K. *Global and Regional Trends in Production, Trade and Consumption of Food Legume Crops*; Michigan State University: East Lansing, MI, USA, 2011.
17. Lovato, F.; Kowaleski, J.; Silva, S.Z.; Heldt, L.F.S. Composição centesimal e conteúdo mineral de diferentes cultivares de feijão biorfortificado (*Phaseolus vulgaris* L.). *Brazilian J. Food Technol.* **2018**, *21*, 1–6. [CrossRef]
18. Suliburska, J.; Krejpcio, Z. Evaluation of the content and bioaccessibility of iron, zinc, calcium and magnesium from groats, rice, leguminous grains and nuts. *J. Food Sci. Technol.* **2014**, *51*, 589–594. [CrossRef] [PubMed]
19. Pereira, E.J.; Carvalho, L.M.; Dellamora-Ortiz, G.M.; Cardoso, F.S.; Carvalho, J.L. Effect of different home-cooking methods on the bioaccessibility of zinc and iron in conventionally bred cowpea (*Vigna unguiculata* L. Walp) consumed in Brazil. *Food Nutr. Res.* **2016**, *60*, 1–6. [CrossRef] [PubMed]
20. Petry, N.; Boy, E.; Wirth, J.P.; Hurrell, R.F. The potential of the common bean (*Phaseolus vulgaris*) as a vehicle for iron biofortification. *Nutrients* **2015**, *7*, 1144–1173. [CrossRef] [PubMed]
21. Companhia Nacional de Abastecimento (Conab), *A Cultura do Feijão, 2018*; Conab: Brasília, Brazil, 2018; ISBN 978 85 60223-12 9. Available online: http://www.conab.gov.br (accessed on 19 July 2018).
22. Institute Medicine (US) Panel on Micronutrients. Dietary Reference Intakes for Vitamin A, Vitamin K, Arsenic, Boron, Chromium, Copper, Iodine, Iron, Manganese, Molybdenum, Nickel, Silicon, Vanadium, and Zinc. Available online: https://www.ncbi.nlm.nih.gov/books/NBK222312/ (accessed on 8 March 2018).
23. Gupta, R.K.; Gangoliya, S.S.; Singh, N.K. Reduction of phytic acid and enhancement of bioavailable micronutrients in food grains. *J. Food Sci. Technol.* **2015**, *52*, 676–684. [CrossRef] [PubMed]
24. Gibson, R.S.; Bailey, K.B.; Gibbs, M.; Ferguson, E.L. A review of phytate, iron, zinc, and calcium concentrations in plant-based complementary foods used in low-income countries and implications for bioavailability. *Food Nutr. Bull.* **2010**, *31*, 134–146. [CrossRef] [PubMed]
25. Kumar, V.; Sinha, A.K.; Makkar, H.P.S.; Becker, K. Dietary roles of phytate and phytase in human nutrition: A review. *Food Chem.* **2010**, *120*, 945–959. [CrossRef]
26. Pedrosa, M.M.; Cuadrado, C.; Burbano, C.; Allaf, K.; Haddad, J.; Gelencsér, E.; Takács, K.; Guillamón, E.; Muzquiz, M. Effect of instant controlled pressure drop on the oligosaccharides, inositol phosphates, trypsin inhibitors and lectins contents of different legumes. *Food Chem.* **2012**, *131*, 862–868. [CrossRef]
27. Fernandes, A.C.; Nishida, W.; Da Costa Proença, R.P. Influence of soaking on the nutritional quality of common beans (*Phaseolus vulgaris* L.) cooked with or without the soaking water: A review. *Int. J. Food Sci. Technol.* **2010**, *45*, 2209–2218. [CrossRef]
28. Ghavidel, R.A.; Prakash, J. The impact of germination and dehulling on nutrients, antinutrients, *In Vitro* iron and calcium bioavailability and *In Vitro* starch and protein digestibility of some legume seeds. *LWT-Food Sci. Technol.* **2007**, *40*, 1292–1299. [CrossRef]
29. Petry, N.; Egli, I.; Zeder, C.; Walczyk, T.; Hurrell, R. Polyphenols and Phytic Acid Contribute to the Low Iron Bioavailability from Common Beans in Young Women. *J. Nutr.* **2010**, *140*, 1977–1982. [CrossRef] [PubMed]
30. Singh, B.; Singh, J.P.; Shevkani, K.; Singh, N.; Kaur, A. Bioactive constituents in pulses and their health benefits. *J. Agric. Food Chem.* **2017**, *57*, 4754–4764. [CrossRef] [PubMed]
31. Ganesan, K.; Xu, B. A critical review on polyphenols and health benefits of black soybeans. *Nutrients* **2017**, *9*, 455. [CrossRef] [PubMed]
32. Ramírez-Jiménez, A.K.; Reynoso-Camacho, R.; Tejero, M.E.; León-Galván, F.; Loarca-Piña, G. Potential role of bioactive compounds of *Phaseolus vulgaris* L. on lipid-lowering mechanisms. *Food Res. Int.* **2015**, *76*, 92–104. [CrossRef]
33. Hart, J.J.; Tako, E.; Kochian, L.V.; Glahn, R.P. Identification of black bean (*Phaseolus vulgaris* L.) polyphenols that inhibit and promote iron uptake by Caco-2 cells. *J. Agric. Food Chem.* **2015**, *63*, 5950–5956. [CrossRef] [PubMed]
34. Fabbri, A.D.T.; Guy, A.C. A review of the impact of preparation and cooking on the nutritional quality of vegetables and legumes. *Int. J. Gastronomy Food Sci.* **2016**, *3*, 2–11. [CrossRef]
35. Feitosa, S.; Korn, M.G.; Pinelli, M.; Oliveira, T.; Boffo, E.; Greiner, R.; Almeida, D.T. Content of Minerals and Antinutritional Factors in Akara (Fried Cowpea Food). *Int. J. Food Process Technol.* **2015**, *2*, 42–50. [CrossRef]
36. Etcheverry, P.; Grusak, M.A.; Fleige, L.E. Application of *In Vitro* bioaccessibility and bioavailability methods for calcium, carotenoids, folate, iron, magnesium, polyphenols, zinc, and vitamins B6, B12, D and E. *Fron. Physiol.* **2012**, *3*, 317. [CrossRef] [PubMed]
37. Perina, E.F.; Carvalho, C.R.L.; Chiorato, A.F.; Lopes, R.L.T.; Gonçalves, J.G.R.; Carbonell, S.A.M. Technological quality of common bean grains obtained in different growing seasons. *Bragantia* **2014**, *73*, 14–22. [CrossRef]

38. AOAC. *Phytate in Foods, Anion-Exchange Method, No. 986.11*, 15th ed.; Official Methods of Analysis AOAC: Arlington, VA, USA, 1990; pp. 800–801.
39. Menezes-Blackburn, D.; Gabler, S.; Greiner, R. Performance of Seven Commercial Phytases in an *In Vitro* Simulation of Poultry Digestive Tract. *J. Agric. Food Chem.* **2015**, *63*, 6142–6149. [CrossRef] [PubMed]
40. King, H.G.; Health, G.W. The chemical analysis of small samples of leaf material and the relationship between disappearance and composition of leaves. *Pedobiologia* **1967**, *7*, 192–197.
41. Broadhurst, R.B.; Jones, W.J. Analysis of condensed tannins using acidified vanillin. *J. Sci. Food Agric.* **1978**, *29*, 788–792. [CrossRef]
42. Rebellato, A.P.; Bussi, J.; Silva, J.G.S.; Greiner, R.; Steel, C.J.; Pallone, J.A.L. Effect of different iron compounds on rheological and technological parameters as well as bioaccessibility of minerals in whole wheat bread. *Food Res. Int.* **2017**, *94*, 65–71. [CrossRef] [PubMed]
43. Katzenberg, M.A.; Saunders, S.R.; Abonyi, S. Bone Chemistry, Food and History: A Case Study from 19th Century Upper Canada. In *Biogeochemical Approaches to Paleodietary Analysis*; Ambrose, S.H., Katzenberg, M.A., Eds.; Kluwer Academic Publishers: New York, NY, USA, 2002.
44. Quintaes, K.D.; Amaya-Farfan, J.; Tomazini, F.M.; Morgano, M.A.; Mantovani, D.M. Migração de minerais de panelas brasileiras de aço inoxidável, ferro fundido e pedra-sabão (esteatito) para simulantes de alimentos. *Ciência e Tecnologia de Alimentos* **2004**, *24*, 397–402. [CrossRef]
45. Drago, S.R. Chapter 5—Minerals. In *Nutraceutical and Functional Food Components: Effects of Innovative Processing Techniques*; Galanakis, C.M., Ed.; Academic Press: London, UK, 2016; pp. 129–157; ISBN 978-0-12-805257-0.
46. Glahn, R. The use of Caco-2 cells in defining nutrient bioavailability: Application to iron bioavailability of foods. In *Designing Functional Foods*; McClements, D.J., Decker, E.A., Eds.; Elsevier: London, UK, 2009; pp. 340–361.
47. Glahn, R.P.; Wortley, G.M.; South, P.K.; Miller, D.D. Inhibition of iron uptake by phytic acid, tannic acid, and $ZnCl_2$: Studies using an *In Vitro* digestion/Caco-2 cell model. *J. Agric. Food Chem.* **2002**, *50*, 390–395. [CrossRef] [PubMed]

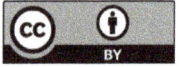

© 2018 by the authors. Licensee MDPI, Basel, Switzerland. This article is an open access article distributed under the terms and conditions of the Creative Commons Attribution (CC BY) license (http://creativecommons.org/licenses/by/4.0/).

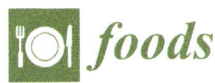

Article

Detection, Purity Analysis, and Quality Assurance of Adulterated Peanut (*Arachis hypogaea*) Oils

Shayla C. Smithson, Boluwatife D. Fakayode, Siera Henderson, John Nguyen and Sayo O. Fakayode *

Department of Physical Sciences, University of Arkansas Fort Smith, 5210 Grand Avenue, P.O. Box 3649, Fort Smith, AR 72913-3649, USA; ssmith10@g.uafs.edu (S.C.S.); Bolufakadami@gmail.com (B.D.F.); shende00@g.uafs.edu (S.H.); jnguye00@g.uafs.edu (J.N.)
* Correspondence: Sayo.Fakayode@uafs.edu; Tel.: +1-479-788-7622; Fax: +1-479-424-6622

Received: 16 June 2018; Accepted: 27 July 2018; Published: 31 July 2018

Abstract: The intake of adulterated and unhealthy oils and trans-fats in the human diet has had negative health repercussions, including cardiovascular disease, causing millions of deaths annually. Sadly, a significant percentage of all consumable products including edible oils are neither screened nor monitored for quality control for various reasons. The prospective intake of adulterated oils and the associated health impacts on consumers is a significant public health safety concern, necessitating the need for quality assurance checks of edible oils. This study reports a simple, fast, sensitive, accurate, and low-cost chemometric approach to the purity analysis of highly refined peanut oils (HRPO) that were adulterated either with vegetable oil (VO), canola oil (CO), or almond oil (AO) for food quality assurance purposes. The Fourier transform infrared spectra of the pure oils and adulterated HRPO samples were measured and subjected to a partial-least-square (PLS) regression analysis. The obtained PLS regression figures-of-merit were incredible, with remarkable linearity (R^2 = 0.994191 or better). The results of the score plots of the PLS regressions illustrate pattern recognition of the adulterated HRPO samples. Importantly, the PLS regressions accurately determined percent compositions of adulterated HRPOs, with an overall root-mean-square-relative-percent-error of 5.53% and a limit-of-detection as low as 0.02% (*wt/wt*). The developed PLS regressions continued to predict the compositions of newly prepared adulterated HRPOs over a period of two months, with incredible accuracy without the need for re-calibration. The accuracy, sensitivity, and robustness of the protocol make it desirable and potentially adoptable by health departments and local enforcement agencies for fast screening and quality assurance of consumable products.

Keywords: peanut-oil; food-analysis; peanut-oil-adulteration; infrared-spectroscopy; partial-least-regression-analysis; food-quality-assurance

1. Introduction

An increase in world population and industrial development has resulted in high demand for consumable products including edible oils. Edible oils are used for domestic cooking, deep frying in fast food restaurants, and for other industrial applications [1,2]. Edible oils are composed of triglyceride molecules, which are required, in certain amounts, in the human diet for energy production and energy storage [3,4]. However, high demand for edible oils such as highly refined peanut oils (HRPOs) has resulted in adulteration of edible oils with cheap, unhealthy, or synthetic oils. Municipalities, health departments, and regulatory agencies, including the United States Food and Drug Administration (FDA), the United State Department of Agriculture, the European Commission, the European Food Safety Authority, and the World Health Organization, are relentless in their efforts to curtail the sales of fake, substandard, and/or adulterated consumable products [5–14]. For instance, efforts have been made by FDA and World Health Organization to prohibit the sale of unhealthy oils and to eliminate trans-fats in the human diet by 2018 and 2023 [15]. Nonetheless, a significant percentage of all consumable products, including edible oils, are neither screened nor monitored for quality control and quality assurance for various and diverging reasons.

Counterfeiting and/or the adulteration of consumable products is even more problematic, rampant, and worrisome in developing countries, where most regulatory agencies lack the infrastructure, skilled inspectors, and/or financial resources to enforce the screening of consumable products. The loopholes and deficiencies in the global monitoring scheme make numerous consumable products highly susceptible to and easy targets for adulteration and/or trafficking. The prospective adulteration of edible oils raises concern about the production of safe edible oils for human consumption. The potential intake of fake and adulterated oils and its associated health impacts are also a nightmare, raising a public health safety concern. For instance, the intake of adulterated and unhealthy oils, and trans-fats in the human diet has had negative health repercussions, including cardiovascular disease, causing millions of deaths annually [15].

To address these concerns, efforts have been devoted to the development of analytical strategies including the use of a high performance liquid chromatography (HPLC), mass spectrometry, electronic nose, isotopic dilution, biomarkers and sensors, nuclear magnetic resonance, deoxyribonucleic acid (DNA) barcoding, and electroanalytical techniques for quality control and assurance of consumable products and edible oils [16–29]. Regardless of the high sensitivity and good accuracy of these techniques, they have inherent challenges and drawbacks such as long analysis times, high cost of instrumentation, and required special training. In addition, some of these methods are not portable, limiting their wider applicability for routine in situ field screening of consumable products. Raman and infrared spectroscopy are non-destructive and rapid techniques that require a small sample size and are capable of solid and liquid sample analysis with little or no sample preparation, making them ideal for fingerprinting, determination of authenticity, and quality assurance of consumable products including edible oils [30–50]. Besides, Raman and infrared spectrometers are portable and fairly inexpensive, allowing affordable and fast in situ field screening of consumable products. Moreover, a combined use of molecular spectroscopy, including Raman, infrared, and fluorescence spectroscopy, and multivariate analyses, has increasingly been used in recent years for sample and instrument calibrations, purity analysis, and quality assurance of consumable products [30–50].

Research from our laboratory [51,52] and from other research laboratories [30–50] has revealed the potential utility of the combined use of molecular spectroscopy and multivariate regression analysis for food purity analysis and quality assurance of adulterated edible oils and essential oils. However, numerous edible oils of high dietary importance and market values such as highly refined peanut oil (HRPO) that are susceptible to adulteration and/or trafficking are yet to be investigated. This study reports a simple, fast, sensitive, accurate, and low-cost chemometric approach to the quality assurance of HRPOs that were adulterated either with edible vegetable oil (VO), canola oil (CO), or almond oil (AO). Specifically, the combined use of Fourier transform infrared spectroscopy (FTIR) and multivariate partial-least-square (PLS) regression for detection, purity analysis, and quality assurance of adulterated HRPOs was investigated.

Peanut oil is derived from the peanut (*Arachis hypogaea*), a legume that is rich in proteins, vitamins, phytochemicals, anti-oxidants, polyphenols, polyunsaturated, and fiber [53–56]. In addition to edible oil production, peanuts have a wide range of other industrial utilities, including the production of peanut butter, peanut flour, animal feed, groundnut cakes, animal protein supplements, and poultry rations [55,57]. The global production of peanut oil is estimated at 5.88 million metric tons in 2018 with multimillion dollar annual global peanut oil sales [55,57]. Highly refined peanut oil is a healthy choice and is widely used for domestic cooking, deep frying in fast foods restaurants, and as salad oils around the world. For instance, Chick-fil-A, one of the leading North American fast-food restaurants, with approximately 2200 restaurants in USA and Canada with $8 billion dollar in revenue, only uses 100% refined peanut oil for all of its cooking and deep frying. Other notable fast-food restaurants including Five Guys, Jimmy Johns, and Subway only use HRPO on their French fries, kettle cooked chips, and carved turkey, respectively. Highly refined peanut oil undergoes several industrial processes including the extraction of protein allergen, discoloration through bleaching, and deodorization [55], making it relatively more expensive than the crude peanut oil. The sale of fake-peanut oil and adulterated HRPO with edible vegetable oils or synthetic oil with a peanut aroma is quite frankly a global challenge, causing economic losses to producers of authentic HRPO.

2. Materials and Methods

2.1. Material and Supplies: Regression Analysis

Highly refined (100%) peanut oil (HRPO) and adulterant vegetable oil (VO), canola oil (CO), and almond oil (AO) were purchased from a local grocery store in Fort Smith, Arkansas, USA.

2.2. Preparation of Adulterated HRPO Samples, FTIR Measurement, PLS Regression, and Multivariate Data Analysis

Twenty-five training sets and calibration samples of adulterated peanut samples were used for each study conducted with vegetable oil, canola oil, and almond oil adulterants. The training set and calibration samples ($n = 25$) of varying compositions of adulterated HRPO with either VO, CO, or AO, ranging from 1–90% (wt/wt), were prepared in sample vials. The samples were kept at room temperature for approximately 48 hours to facilitate homogenization of HRPO and the adulterant oils. The FTIR spectra of the adulterated HRPOs were measured using an ATR-FTIR spectrometer (Thermo Scientific NiCOLET iS5, Waltham, MA, USA). The FTIR spectrum of each sample was scanned 25 times with a resolution of 4 cm^{-1} over a 600 cm^{-1} to 4000 cm^{-1} wavenumber range. Partial-least-regression and chemometric data analysis was performed using the software The Unscrambler (CAMO Software, 9.8, Oslo, Norway).

3. Results and Discussion

3.1. Physical Examination and FTIR Property of Pure and Adulterated HRPO Oils

The initial study involved the physical and FTIR spectroscopic examination of pure edible highly refined peanut oil (HRPO), vegetable oil (VO), canola oil (CO), almond oil (AO), and adulterated HRPOs. Highly refined peanut oil is pale-yellow, with no apparent peanut odor. The physical appearance and the color of pure HRPO, VO, CO, and AO are very similar and indistinguishable. Similarly, the physical appearance, including the color, of pure HRPO and adulterated HRPOs counterparts is identical, making it challenging to use ordinary visual examination for the detection of a suspected adulterated HRPO.

The FTIR spectra of pure HRPO, VO, CO, and AO samples showing the notable and characteristic C–CH_2 asymmetric stretch (C–H) stretching (~2921 cm^{-1}); CH_2 symmetric stretching (C–H) (~2853 cm^{-1}); ester C=O stretching (~1745 cm^{-1}); CH_2 wagging (~1160 cm^{-1}); symmetric H–C–H bending (~1380 cm^{-1}); and CH_2 scissoring (~1460 cm^{-1}) of triglyceride component of HRPO, VO, CO, and AO [32,33] are shown in Figure 1. Expectedly, pure HRPO, VO, CO, and AO have similar FTIR absorption profiles, primarily because all edible oils contain the triglyceride molecules that are responsible for FTIR absorptions [32,33]. Also, edible oils contain triglyceride molecules that are required, in certain amounts, in the human diet for energy production, utility, and energy storage [3,4]. Figure 2 shows the cross sections of FTIR spectra of the training set and calibration samples with varying % composition of HRPO adulterated with VO, CO, and AO adulterants. Although the physical appearance of the pure HRPOs and adulterated HRPOs are indistinguishable, the profile of FTIR spectra of pure HRPO and adulterated HRPO differ and vary with the percentage compositions of the adulterated HRPO samples. The observed variations and changes of FTIR spectra with compositions of adulterated HRPOs is an indicative of interactions of the HRPO with adulterant oils as a result of hydrophobic interactions and/or through hydrogen bonding involving the triglyceride carbonyl group. Differences in the FTIR spectra profile of pure HRPO and adulterated HPPO can, therefore, be used for quick screening for the detection of adulterated peanut oils.

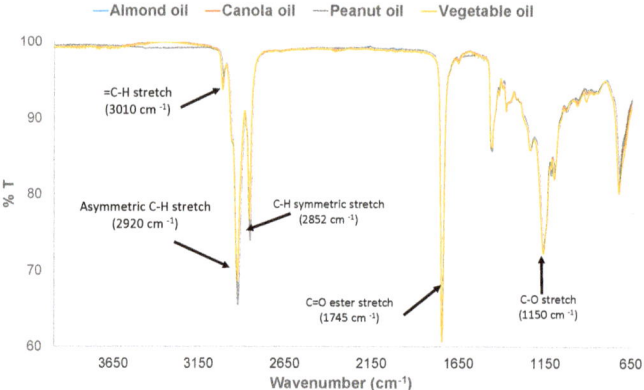

Figure 1. FTIR spectra of pure highly refined peanut oil, vegetable oil (VO), canola oil (CO), and almond oil (AO).

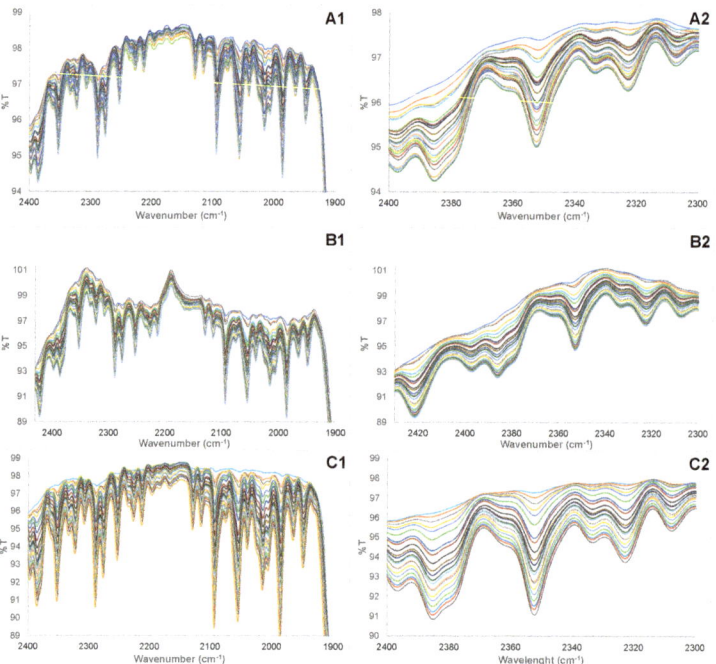

Figure 2. Cross section of FTIR spectra of the training set and calibration samples of: (**A1,A2**) highly refined (100%) peanut oil (HRPO) adulterated with vegetable oil, (**B1,B2**) HRPO adulterated with canola oil, (**C1,C2**) HRPO adulterated with almond oil.

3.2. PLS Regression Modeling

The complexity, variation, and spectral overlapping at multiple wavenumbers observed in Figure 2 preclude the likely use of ordinary visual examination for adulterated HRPO pattern recognition or the use of univariate spectral analysis (spectral analysis at one wavenumber) to achieve any meaningful sample calibrations or regression analysis for purity analysis and determination of percent composition of adulterated HRPO samples. The use of multivariate analysis (spectral analysis over a range of wavenumbers) such as partial-least-square (PLS) is more desirable and capable of complex spectral data analysis for sample calibration. The PLS can capitalize on the changes and variability, such as those observed in Figure 2, to extract the most valuable information that is required for sample calibration and for PLS regression modelling to determine the compositions of adulterated HRPOs. The most valuable information in the spectral data set is invariably accompanied with the directions that contains the most substantial variability. The detailed PLS mathematical expressions have been comprehensively discussed and reported elsewhere [58–62].

Generally speaking, the goal of any PLS regression is to decompose the original data matrix A into two components, a *"structure component"* and a *"noise component"* that can be represented by Equation (1).

$$A = TP^T + E \qquad (1)$$

where A is the original $k \times n$ data matrix of FTIR % transmittance data of adulterated HRPOs in this study, T and P are two new matrices that must be evaluated and determined, and E is a $k \times n$ residual matrix that represents the unexplained variance or *"noise component"* in the model. The *"structure component"* of A is given by TP^T where the superscript T denotes the transpose of P, achievable by substituting rows for columns. Each PLS component is a variance-scaled vector that accounts for a certain amount of variability in the data set.

Partial-least-regression modelling also aims to determine a regression vector, which constitutes the mathematical model that relates the FTIR spectral data in this study to the % compositions of adulterated HRPOs. In the case of a single sample, the relationship between the dependent variable (y-variable, % composition of adulterated HRPOs) and the independent variable (x-variables, the FTIR spectral data) can be expressed mathematically using Equation (2).

$$y_i = b_0 + x_1 b_{i1} + x_2 b_{i2} + x_3 b_{i3} + \ldots \ldots \ldots x_n b_{in} \qquad (2)$$

where y_i is the value of y predicted by the PLS regression model for the ith sample, the b_i are the regression coefficients that constitute the regression vector, and the $x_{i\lambda}$ terms represent the FTIR intensities for the ith sample over the wavenumber index from 1 to n. Equation (2) can further be expressed in matrix notation as shown in Equation (3).

$$Y = Xb \qquad (3)$$

where Y contains the matrix values of the dependent variables for all samples, X is a matrix composed of values of the independent variables of all samples, and b contains the regression vector. As soon as a regression model has been established and optimized, it can be utilized to calculate y_i for any series of unknown samples exclusively from their spectra using Equation (3).

The predictive ability of any PLS regression model for the y-variable invariably relies on the assumption of no co-linearity among the x-variables, which is an invalid assumption for a PLS regression involving spectral data analysis. Hence, the initial task in any PLS regression modeling is to carefully eliminate any inherent co-linearity in the spectral data or x-variables. Removal of co-linearity among x-variables is achievable by transforming the original data matrix **A** from the initial xyz-coordinate system (made up of n variables) into a new variance-scaled eigenvector coordinate system with fewer variables, where each new variable is orthogonal to the others. The use of PLS is desirable because it reduces the data dimensionality from n to a significantly smaller value.

Additionally, the actual number of vectors required to construct the new variable space is adjustable to fit the expected *"noise"* level of the original data matrix **A**. The new variance-scaled eigenvector coordinate system is thus composed of a smaller number of orthogonal vectors known as the partial least square (PLS) component. The first PLS component of a dataset usually accounts for most of variance in the data. Each successive PLS component accounts for a lesser variance in the dataset. Therefore, only a few PLS components often contain the most valuable information in a dataset. After the first few PLS components are evaluated and determined, the remaining variance is summed together into the **E** matrix (noise component) that is not accounted for by the PLS model is eliminated.

3.3. Figures-of-Merit of PLS Regression Model, Limit-of-Detection (LOD), and Limit-of-Quantitation (LOQ)

The result of the PLS regression models developed for adulterated HRPOs using VO, CO, and AO adulterants using a full cross validation is shown in Figure 3. In Figure 3, plots A1, A2, and A3 illustrate the regression coefficients as a function of wavenumber for the PLS regression models constructed for adulterated HRPO with VO, CO, and AO adulterant, respectively. The contribution of the magnitude of the coefficients according to wavenumber varies widely. Some wavenumbers contributed positively to the PLS regression, while other wavenumbers contributed negatively to the PLS regression model. The *score plot* of PLS1 versus PLS2 is shown in Figure 3B. The number of the adulterated HRPO samples ($n = 25$ in this study) used for the training set and calibration samples is small in comparison with the FTIR spectral data points (>3600). In theory ($n - 1$), PLSs can be used for data analysis, therefore 24-PLSs can be used in this study. However, the first two PLSs accounted for 100% of the variability in the FTIR spectral data (x-variable) and 97% of the percent composition of adulterated HRPO samples. Thus, 2-PLS components are appropriate to represent the data, thereby significantly reducing the data dimensionality. Interestingly, the *score plots* of PLS showed the grouping of the adulterated HRPO samples into two notable and different categories. The samples containing higher percent compositions of VO in the adulterated HRPOs were conspicuously grouped on the right hand side corner (first and second quadrants) of the *score plot*. In contrast, the samples containing higher percent compositions of HRPO in the adulterated samples were grouped on the left hand side (third and fourth quadrants) of the *score plot*. Figure 3(C1) shows the plot of the actual versus the percent compositions of adulterated HRPO with VO determined by the PLS regression. Obviously, the predicted percentage compositions of adulterated HRPO samples favorably compared with the actual percentage composition of adulterated HRPO of the training set and calibration samples. The outcomes of the PLS regression including the *score plot* of the adulterated HRPO with CO and AO adulterants showed similar pattern recognition data.

A summary of the developed PLS regression models figures-of-merit including the square correlation coefficients (R^2), limits-of-detection (*LOD*), and limits-of-quantification (*LOQ*), are shown in Table 1. The figures-of-merit of the PLS regressions were incredible, with remarkable linearity ($R^2 = 0.994191$ or better). The *LOD* and *LOQ* values were calculated as 3 s/m and 10 s/m, respectively, where s is the standard deviation of the FTIR intensity of the blanks and m is the slope of the PLS regression calibration curve. The *LOD* ranged between 0.02% wt/wt for HRPO adulterated with CO and 0.27 % wt/wt for HRPO adulterated with VO, demonstrate the capability of the developed PLS regressions for detection of adulterated HRPO at low levels of adulteration.

Table 1. Figures-of-merit of partial least squares (PLS) regression calibration curves.

	Wavenumber (cm^{-1})	Offset	Slope	R^2	LOD (%wt/wt)	LOQ (%wt/wt)
HRPO-VO	2235–3300	0.572672	0.988415	0.994191	0.27%	0.90
HRPO-CO	2235–3300	0.075944	0.998477	0.999238	0.02%	0.05
HRPO-AO	400–4000	0.154691	0.996644	0.998321	0.02%	0.07

R^2—*correlation coefficients; LOD—limits-of-detection; LOQ—limits-of-quantification. HRPO—highly refined (100%) peanut oil; VO—vegetable oil; CO—canola oil; AO—almond oil.*

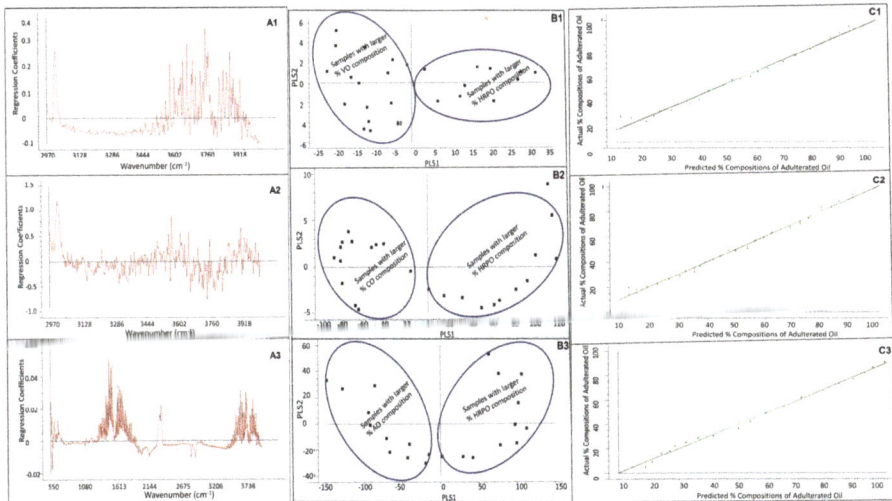

Figure 3. Summary of the partial least square (PLS) regression: (**A1**) regression coefficient of PLS versus wavenumber of HRPO adulterated with vegetable oil; (**A2**) regression coefficient of PLS versus wavenumber of HRPO adulterated with canola oil; (**A3**) regression coefficient of PLS versus wavenumber of HRPO adulterated with almond oil; (**B1**) score plot of PLS regression of HRPO adulterated with vegetable oil; (**B2**) score plot of PLS regression of HRPO adulterated with canola oil; (**B3**) score plot of PLS regression of HRPO adulterated with almond oil; (**C1**) plot of predicted versus actual composition of HRPO adulterated with vegetable oil; (**C2**) plot of predicted versus actual composition of HRPO adulterated with canola oil; (**C3**) plot of predicted versus actual composition of HRPO adulterated with almond oil.

3.4. Determination of Percentage Compositions of Adulterated HRPO Samples

The validation studies were conducted to assess the performance and predictive ability of the PLS regression models for the determination of the percent composition of adulterated HRPO samples. Twenty (22) validation samples each were used for HRPOs that were adulterated with VO and CO. However, 21 validation samples were used for HRPOs adulterated with AO. The FTIR spectra of the adulterated HRPO validation samples using VO, CO, and AO adulterants are shown in Figure 4. It must be highlighted that while the range of the percent compositions of adulterated HRPO in the training set and validation samples are the same, the compositions of adulterated HRPO of the training set and validation samples are totally autonomous. The summary of the results of the validation study conducted for adulterated HRPO showing the actual and the determined compositions of adulterated HRPOs using VO, CO, and AO adulterants are shown in Tables 2–4, respectively. The obtained low percent relative error (%RE) of the determined compositions of adulterated HRPOs obviously demonstrates the accuracy of the protocol. The predictive ability of the PLS regression model was further assessed by root-mean-square-relative-percent-errors (*RMS%RE*) for the determination of percent compositions of adulterated HRPOs. The PLS regression models determined percent compositions of adulterated HRPO with VO, CO, and AO with low *RMS%RE* of determination of 2.77%, 5.51%, and 8.32%, respectively, with an overall average *RMS%RE* of 5.53%.

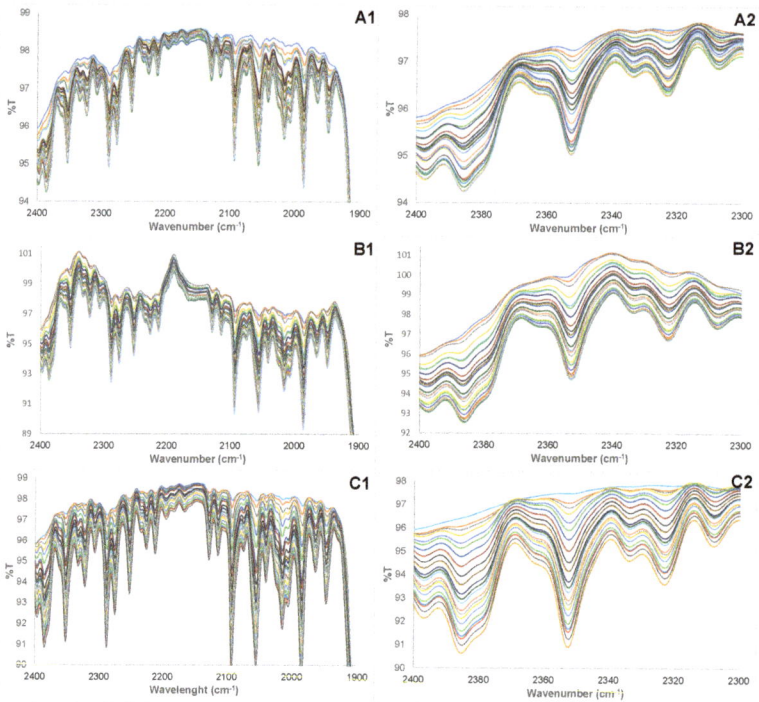

Figure 4. Cross section of FTIR spectra of validation samples of the following: (**A1,A2**) HRPO adulterated with vegetable oil, (**B1,B2**) HRPO adulterated with canola oil, (**C1,C2**) HRPO adulterated with almond oil.

Table 2. Validation conducted for highly refined peanut oil (HRPO) adulterated with vegetable oil (VO).

Sample	% HRPO Predicted	Actual % HRPO	%RE	% VO Predicted	Actual % VO	%RE
V1	90.8	89.1	−1.95	9.2	10.9	15.9
V2	85.6	85.1	−0.58	14.4	14.9	3.30
V3	82.5	82.4	−0.07	17.5	17.6	0.33
V4	77.8	79.1	1.63	22.2	20.9	−6.19
V5	72.0	74.0	2.62	28.0	26.0	−7.45
V6	69.2	69.8	0.88	30.8	30.2	−2.02
V7	63.8	64.4	1.04	36.3	35.6	−1.88
V8	61.1	60.4	−1.12	38.9	39.6	1.72
V9	56.5	57.7	1.98	43.5	42.3	−2.69
V10	56.0	54.4	−2.90	44.0	45.6	3.47
V11	52.2	51.6	−1.06	47.8	48.4	1.13
V12	49.3	48.4	−1.96	50.7	51.6	1.84
V13	46.2	45.1	−2.51	53.8	54.9	2.06
V14	43.0	42.7	−0.87	57.0	57.3	0.65
V15	38.6	39.7	2.53	61.4	60.3	−1.66
V16	37.0	37.8	1.94	63.0	62.2	−1.18
V17	34.5	35.8	3.67	65.5	64.2	−2.04
V18	31.4	32.8	4.29	68.6	67.2	−2.09
V19	27.7	29.7	6.76	72.3	70.3	−2.85
V20	27.2	27.2	−0.23	72.8	72.8	0.09
V21	22.9	23.5	2.51	77.1	76.5	−0.77
V22	19.6	20.8	5.79	80.4	79.2	−1.52
RMS%RE			2.77			4.37

RE—relative error.

Table 3. Validation conducted for highly refined peanut oil (HRPO) adulterated with canola oil (CO).

Sample	% HPPO Predicted	Actual % HPPO	%RE	% CO Predicted	Actual % CO	%RE
V1	89.8	87.9	−2.07	10.2	12.1	15.1
V2	84.0	84.3	0.37	16.0	15.7	−2.01
V3	80.2	82.7	2.96	19.8	17.3	−14.1
V4	77.9	77.2	−0.91	22.1	22.8	3.08
V5	71.0	74.0	4.03	29.0	26.0	−11.5
V6	68.7	70.8	3.00	31.3	29.2	−7.29
V7	63.7	64.3	1.04	36.3	35.7	−1.88
V8	60.5	61.1	0.88	39.5	38.9	−1.38
V9	55.5	58.0	4.36	44.5	42.0	−6.03
V10	54.6	56.0	2.45	45.4	44.0	0.12
V11	51.5	51.2	−0.68	48.5	48.8	0.71
V12	49.4	48.4	−2.09	50.6	51.6	1.96
V13	46.2	46.4	0.38	53.8	53.6	−0.33
V14	46.3	43.5	−6.45	53.7	56.5	4.97
V15	40.0	41.0	2.31	60.0	59.0	−1.61
V16	37.7	38.5	1.98	62.3	61.5	−1.24
V17	33.8	36.9	8.47	66.2	63.1	−4.96
V18	32.8	34.4	4.64	67.2	65.6	−2.43
V19	29.6	31.5	5.89	70.4	68.5	−2.70
V20	26.3	28.6	8.07	73.7	71.4	−3.23
V21	26.0	25.0	−3.96	74.0	75.0	1.32
V22	20.8	20.9	0.66	79.2	79.1	−0.17
RMS%RE			5.51			5.87

Table 4. Validation conducted for highly refined peanut oil (HRPO) adulterated with almond oil (AO).

Sample	% HRPO Predicted	Actual % HRPO	%RE	% AO Predicted	Actual % AO	%RE
V1	89.6	88.3	−1.50	10.4	11.7	11.3
V2	85.7	85.9	0.24	14.3	14.1	−1.44
V3	82.3	83.7	1.66	17.7	16.3	−8.54
V4	77.9	79.8	2.45	22.1	20.2	−9.71
V5	76.0	76.7	0.89	24.0	23.3	−2.92
V6	70.3	71.4	1.51	29.7	28.6	−3.76
V7	62.1	64.9	4.25	37.9	35.1	−7.85
V8	58.4	58.7	0.43	41.6	41.3	−0.62
V9	51.3	51.8	0.99	48.7	48.2	−1.06
V10	46.3	44.4	−4.17	53.7	55.6	3.33
V11	39.8	42.5	6.47	60.2	57.5	−4.79
V12	37.3	36.9	−0.97	62.7	63.1	0.57
V13	34.1	33.0	−3.56	65.9	67.0	1.75
V14	28.1	29.4	4.22	71.9	70.6	−1.75
V15	28.1	23.2	−20.77	71.9	76.8	6.29
V16	23.5	20.9	−12.34	76.5	79.1	3.27
V17	21.2	17.7	−19.46	78.8	82.3	4.19
V18	16.8	16.3	−3.13	83.2	83.7	0.61
V19	14.2	14.7	3.42	85.8	85.3	−0.59
V20	11.5	12.3	6.51	88.5	87.7	−0.91
V21	8.3	10.0	17.42	91.7	90.0	−1.95
RMS%RE			8.32			4.86

Although AO is relatively more expensive than HRPO, our study has demonstrated that the purity, authenticity, and percent compositions of adulterated HRPOs can be accurately determined regardless of the edible oil used as adulterant. It must be highlighted that our protocol was not only capable of determining the percentage composition of HRPO in adulterated HRPOs with AO with good accuracy, but it was also capable of determination of the compositions of AO in the adulterated HRPOs with an *RMS%RE* of 4.86% (Table 4). This capability is commendable and appealing, demonstrating the extensive applicability of the protocol for purity analysis of a wide range of edible oils of high dietary and market values.

In order to assess the robustness and reliability of the developed PLS regressions for the determination of percent compositions of future samples of adulterated HRPOs, a set of newly prepared adulterated HRPO samples was prepared over a period of two months. The FTIR spectra of the samples were collected and the originally developed PLS regressions were used to predict the percent compositions of adulterated HRPOs. Interestingly, the developed PLS regression models continued to predict the compositions of newly prepared adulterated HRPOs over a period of two months with incredible accuracy without the need for re-calibration, indicating the robustness of the protocol for purity analysis of adulterated HRPOs.

The result of the study is adoptable and can possibly be used by municipal health departments and local enforcement agencies for rapid, in situ, and field screening of a suspected adulterated HRPO. For instance, the FTIR spectra of pure and adulterated HRPOs can be collected and stored in the database. Hand-held IR spectrometers can be used in situ on the field to rapidly obtain an IR spectrum of a suspected adulterated HRPO. The FTIR spectrum profile of a suspected adulterated HRPO can then be compared with the FTIR spectrum of the adulterated HRPO in the database for similarities or differences. The obtained FTIR spectrum of the adulterated HRPO can be subjected to PLS regression on a laptop computer in the field and optimized. The location of the suspected adulterated HRPOs on the PLS regression *score plot* can be further used for rapid pattern recognition. The developed PLS regression can subsequently be used for purity analysis of the suspected adulterated HRPO samples on the field.

4. Conclusions

The result of the combined use of Fourier transform infrared spectroscopy and multivariate partial-least-square (PLS) regression models for rapid purity analysis of highly refined peanut oils (HRPO) that were adulterated with either vegetable oil (VO), canola oil (CO), or almond oil (AO) for food quality assurance purposes is reported. The figures-of-merit of the PLS regression models were incredible with desirable linearity, sensitivity, and robustness. The results of the score plots of the PLS regressions illustrate pattern recognition of the adulterated HRPO samples. The PLS regression models determined compositions of adulterated HRPO with excellent accuracy and low-detection-limits, allowing detection of adulterated HRPO in small quantities. Most importantly, the developed PLS regression models continued to predict the compositions of newly prepared adulterated HRPOs over a period of two months with incredible accuracy without the need for re-calibration, indicating the robustness of the protocol for purity analysis of adulterated HRPOs. The low-cost, non-destructive property; the small sample requirement, high accuracy, and sensitivity; and the simplicity of the protocol make it appealing for quick, in situ, and field screening of suspected adulterated oils by municipalities, health departments, and local enforcement agencies for quality assurance and safety of consumable products.

Author Contributions: Conceptualization, S.O.F. is the project administrator and supervisor. S.O.F. conceptualized the research idea, performed the multivariate regression analysis, and was involved in manuscript preparation and edit. S.C.S., B.D.F., S.H., and J.N. performed the experimental sample preparation and infrared instrumental measurement, preparation of graphs and data analysis.

Funding: This research received no external funding.

Acknowledgments: The assistant of Brianda Elzey and David Pollard for manuscript proofreading is acknowledged.

Conflicts of Interest: The authors declare that there is no conflict of interest in this study.

References

1. O'Brien, R.D. *Fats and Oils: Formulating and Processing for Applications*; CRC Press: Boca Raton, FL, USA, 2004; pp. 1–147.

2. Majchrzak, T.; Wojnowski, W.; Dymerski, T.; Gebicki, J.; Namies'nik, J. Electronic noses in classification and quality control of edible oils: A review. *Food Chem.* **2018**, *246*, 192–201. [CrossRef] [PubMed]
3. Yang, Y.; Zhang, L.; Li, P.; Yu, L.; Mao, J.; Wang, X.; Zhang, Q. A review of chemical composition and nutritional properties of minor vegetable oils in China. *Trends Food Sci. Technol.* **2018**, *74*, 26–32. [CrossRef]
4. Dorni, C.; Sharma, P.; Saikia, G.; Longvah, T. Fatty acid profile of edible oils and fats consumed in India. *Food Chem.* **2018**, *238*, 9–15. [CrossRef] [PubMed]
5. Lutter, R. Addressing Challenges of Economically-Motivated Adulteration. Presented at Public Meeting on Economically Motivated Adulteration, College Park, MD, USA, 06 April. *Fed. Regist.* **2009**, *74*, 15497–15499.
6. Everstine, K.; Spink, J.; Kennedy, S. Analysis of Food Fraud and Economically Motivated Adulteration incidents. *J. Food Prot.* **2013**, *4*, 560–735.
7. Spink, J.; Moyer, D.C. Understanding and combating food fraud. *Food Technol.* **2013**, *67*, 30–35.
8. European Commission. Commission Decision of 12 August 2002 implementing Council Directive 96/23/EC concerning the performance of analytical methods and the interpretation of results (2002/657/EC). *Off. J. Eur. Commun.* **2002**, *221*, 8–36.
9. European Commission. Food Fraud. 2006. Available online: http://ec.europa.eu/food/safety/official_controls/food_fraud/index_en.htm (accessed on 4 June 2018).
10. European Food Safety Authority. Regulation (EC) No 178/2002 of the European Parliament and of the Council of 28 January 2002 laying down the general principles and requirements of food law, establishing the European Food Safety Authority and laying down procedures in matters of food safety. *Off. J. Eur. Commun.* **2002**, *31*, 1–24.
11. European Parliament. EP Report 2013/2091(INI). *Report on the Food Crisis, Fraud in the Food Chain and the Control Thereof*. European Parliament—Committee on the Environment, Public Health and Food Safety. 4 December 2013. Available online: http://www.europarl.europa.eu/sides/getDoc.do?pubRef=-//EP//TEXT+REPORT+A7-2013-0434+0+DOC+XML+V0//EN (accessed on 4 June 2018).
12. Johnson, R. *Food Fraud and "Economically Motivated Adulteration of Food and Food Ingredients"*. Congressional Research Service: 10 January 2014. Available online: https://fas.org/sgp/crs/misc/R43358.pdf (accessed on 5 June 2018).
13. Wheatley, V.; Spink, J. Defining the public health threat of dietary supplement fraud. *Compr. Rev. Food Sci. Food Saf.* **2013**, *12*, 599–613. [CrossRef]
14. U.S. Pharmacopeial Convention. USP's Food Fraud Database. Available online: https://www.foodfraud.org/ (accessed on 4 June 2018).
15. Tavernise, S. The New York Times: FDA Set 2018 Deadline to Rid Foods of Trans Fats. Available online: https://www.nytimes.com/2015/06/17/health/fda-gives-food-industry-three-years-eliminate-trans-fats.html (accessed on 15 May 2018).
16. Miele, M.M.; Anderson, S.L.; Blackburn, S.C.; Bradley, S.L.; Craft, D.L.; Flynn, C.J.; Fulton, T.J.; Rovnyak, D. NMR Characterization of Adulterants in Health Supplements. *Chem. Educ.* **2016**, *21*, 139–142.
17. Parveen, I.; Gafner, S.; Techen, N.; Murch, S.J.; Khan, I.A. DNA barcoding for the identification of botanicals in herbal medicine and dietary supplements: Strengths and limitations. *Planta Med.* **2016**, *82*, 1225–1235. [CrossRef] [PubMed]
18. Reid, L.M.; O'Donnell, C.P.; Downey, G. Recent technological advances for the determination of food authenticity. *Trends Food Sci. Technol.* **2006**, *17*, 344–353. [CrossRef]
19. Wielogorska, E.; Chevallier, O.; Black, C.; Galvin-King, P.; Delêtre, M.; Kelleher, C.T.; Haughey, S.A.; Elliott, C.T. Development of a comprehensive analytical platform for the detection and quantitation of food fraud using a biomarker approach. The oregano adulteration case study. *Food Chem.* **2018**, *239*, 32–39. [CrossRef] [PubMed]
20. Cornet, V.; Govaert, Y.; Moens, G.; Van Loco, J.; Degroodt, J.M. Development of a Fast Analytical Method for the Determination of Sudan Dyes in Chili- and Curry-Containing Foodstuffs by High-Performance Liquid Chromatography—Photodiode Array Detection. *J. Agric. Food Chem.* **2006**, *54*, 639–644. [CrossRef] [PubMed]
21. Ruf, J.; Walter, P.; Kandler, H.; Kaufmann, A. Discovery and structural elucidation of the illegal azo dye Basic Red 46 in sumac spice. *J. Food Addit. Contam.* **2012**, *29*, 897–907. [CrossRef] [PubMed]
22. Marieschi, M.; Torelli, A.; Beghé, D.; Bruni, R. Authentication of *Punica granatum* L.: Development of SCAR markers for the detection of 10 fruits potentially used in economically motivated adulteration. *Food Chem.* **2016**, *202*, 438–444. [CrossRef] [PubMed]

23. Wang, S.; Guo, Q.; Wang, L.; Lin, L.; Shi, H.; Cao, H.; Cao, B. Detection of honey adulteration with starch syrup by high performance liquid chromatography. *Food Chem.* **2015**, *172*, 669–674. [CrossRef] [PubMed]
24. Domingues, D.S.; Pauli, E.D.; de Abreu, J.E.M.; Massura, F.W.; Cristiano, V.; Santos, M.J.; Nixdorf, S.L. Detection of roasted and ground coffee adulteration by HPLC by amperometric and by post-column derivatization UV–Vis detection. *Food Chem.* **2014**, *146*, 353–362. [CrossRef] [PubMed]
25. Apetrei, I.M.; Apetrei, C. Detection of virgin olive oil adulteration using a voltammetric e-tongue. *Comput. Electron. Agric.* **2014**, *108*, 148–154. [CrossRef]
26. Ribeiro, R.O.R.; Mársico, E.T.; Carneiro, C.D.S.; Monteiro, M.L.G.; Conte Júnior, C.; de Jesus, E.F.O. Detection of honey adulteration of high fructose corn syrup by Low Field Nuclear Magnetic Resonance (LF ^{1}H NMR). *J. Food Eng.* **2014**, *135*, 39–43. [CrossRef]
27. Fang, G.; Goh, J.Y.; Tay, M.; Lau, H.F.; Li, S.F.Y. Characterization of oils and fats by ^{1}H NMR and GC/MS fingerprinting: Classification, prediction and detection of adulteration. *Food Chem.* **2013**, *138*, 1461–1469. [CrossRef] [PubMed]
28. Zhu, W.; Wang, X.; Chen, L. Rapid detection of peanut oil adulteration using low-field nuclear magnetic resonance and chemometrics. *Food Chem.* **2017**, *216*, 268–274. [CrossRef] [PubMed]
29. Zhang, L.; Li, P.; Sun, X.; Wang, X.; Xu, B.; Wang, X.; Ding, X. Classification and adulteration detection of vegetable oils based on fatty acid profiles. *J. Agric. Food Chem.* **2014**, *62*, 8745–8751. [CrossRef] [PubMed]
30. Guillen, M.D.; Cabo, N. Infrared Spectroscopy in the Study of Edible Oils and Fats. *J. Sci. Food Agric.* **1997**, *75*, 1–11. [CrossRef]
31. Muik, B.; Lendl, B.; Molina-Diaz, A.; Valcarcel, M.; Ayora-Canada, M.J. Two-dimensional correlation spectroscopy and multivariate curve resolution for the study of lipid oxidation in edible oils monitored by FTIR and FT-Raman spectroscopy. *Anal. Chim. Acta* **2007**, *593*, 54–67. [CrossRef] [PubMed]
32. Rodrigues Júnior, P.H.; de Sá Oliveira, K.; de Almeida, C.E.; De Oliveira, L.F.; Stephani, R.; Pinto Mda, S.; de Carvalho, A.F.; Perrone, Í.T. FT-Raman and chemometric tools for rapid determination of quality parameters in milk powder: Classification of samples for the presence of lactose and fraud detection byaddition of maltodextrin. *Food Chem.* **2016**, *196*, 584–588. [CrossRef] [PubMed]
33. Ding, X.; Ni, Y.; Kokot, S. NIR spectroscopy and chemometrics for the discrimination of pure, powdered, purple sweet potatoes and their samples adulterated with the white sweet potato flour. *Chemom. Intell. Lab. Syst.* **2015**, *144*, 17–23. [CrossRef]
34. Kurniawati, E.; Rohman, A.; Triyana, K. Analysis of lard in meatball broth using Fourier transform infrared spectroscopy and chemometrics. *Meat Sci.* **2014**, *96*, 94–98. [CrossRef] [PubMed]
35. Li, B.; Wang, H.; Zhao, Q.; Ouyang, J.; Wu, Y. Rapid detection of authenticity and adulteration of walnut oil by FTIR and fluorescence spectroscopy: A comparative study. *Food Chem.* **2015**, *181*, 25–30. [CrossRef] [PubMed]
36. De Sá Oliveira, K.; Callegaro, L.S.; Stephani, R.; Almeida, M.R.; Oliveira, L.F.C. Analysis of spreadable cheese by Raman spectroscopy and chemometric tools. *Food Chem.* **2016**, *194*, 441–446. [CrossRef] [PubMed]
37. Nekvapil, F.; Brezestean, I.; Barchewitz, D.; Glamuzina, B.; Chiş, V.; Pinzaru, S.C. Citrus fruits freshness assessment using Raman spectroscopy. *Food Chem.* **2018**, *242*, 560–567. [CrossRef] [PubMed]
38. Alvarenga Junior, B.R.; Soares, F.L.F.; Ardila, J.A.; Durango, L.G.C.; Forim, M.R.; Carneiro, R.L. Determination of B-complex vitamins in pharmaceutical formulations by surface-enhanced Raman spectroscopy. *Spectrochim. Acta Mol. Biomol. Spectrosc.* **2018**, *188*, 589–595. [CrossRef] [PubMed]
39. Martin, C.; Bruneel, J.; Guyon, F.; Médina, B.; Jourdes, M.; Teissedre, P.; Guillaume, F. Raman spectroscopy of white wines. *Food Chem.* **2015**, *181*, 235–240. [CrossRef] [PubMed]
40. Mandrile, A.M.; Giovannozzi, F.; Durbiano, G.; Martrab, A.M. Rossi. Rapid and sensitive detection of pyrimethanil residues on pome fruits by Surface Enhanced Raman Scattering. *Food Chem.* **2018**, *244*, 16–24. [CrossRef] [PubMed]
41. Trebolazabala, J.; Maguregui, M.; Morillas, H.; Diego, A.; Madariaga, J.M. Portable Raman spectroscopy for an in-situ monitoring the ripening of tomato (*Solanum lycopersicum*) fruits. *Spectrochim. Acta Mol. Biomol. Spectrosc.* **2017**, *180*, 138–143. [CrossRef] [PubMed]
42. Lipiäinen, I.; Fraser-Miller, S.J.; Gordon, K.C.; Strachan, C.J. Direct comparison of low- and mid-frequency Raman spectroscopy for quantitative solid-state pharmaceutical analysis. *J. Pharm. Biomed. Anal.* **2018**, *149*, 343–350. [CrossRef] [PubMed]

43. Chen, D.; Xie, X.; Ao, H.; Liu, J.; Peng, C. Raman spectroscopy in quality control of Chinese herbal medicine. *J. Chin. Med. Assoc.* **2017**, *80*, 288–296. [CrossRef] [PubMed]
44. Mandrile, L.; Amato, G.; Marchis, D.; Martra, G.; Rossi, A.M. Species-specific detection of processed animal proteins in feed by Raman Spectroscopy. *Food Chem.* **2017**, *229*, 268–275. [CrossRef] [PubMed]
45. Nedeljkovic, A.; Tomasevic, I.; Miocinovic, J.; Pudja, P. Feasibility of discrimination of dairy creams and cream-like analogues using Raman spectroscopy and chemometric analysis. *Food Chem.* **2017**, *232*, 487–492. [CrossRef] [PubMed]
46. Li, Y.; Fang, T.; Zhu, S.; Huang, F.; Chen, Z.; Wang, Y. Detection of olive oil adulteration with waste cooking oil via Raman spectroscopy combined with iPLS and SiPLS. *Spectrochim. Acta Mol. Biomol. Spectrosc.* **2018**, *189*, 37–43. [CrossRef] [PubMed]
47. Gao, F.; Xu, L.; Zhang, Y.; Yang, Z.; Han, L.; Liu, X. Analytical Raman spectroscopic study for discriminant analysis of different animal-derived foodstuffs. Understanding the hug Muik correlation between Raman spectroscopy and lipid characteristics. *Food Chem.* **2018**, *240*, 989–996. [CrossRef] [PubMed]
48. Sebben, J.A.; Espindola, J.S.; Ranzan, L.; Moura, N.F.; Trierweiler, L.F.; Trierweiler, J.O. Development of a quantitative approach using Raman spectroscopy for carotenoids determination in processed sweet potato. *Food Chem.* **2018**, *245*, 1224–1231. [CrossRef] [PubMed]
49. Feudjio, W.M.; Ghalila, H.; Nsangou, M.; Majdi, Y.; Kongbonga, Y.M. Fluorescence Spectroscopy Combined with Chemometrics for the Investigation of the Adulteration of Essential Oils. *Food Anal. Method* **2017**, *10*, 2539–2548. [CrossRef]
50. Ellis, D.I.; Brewster, V.L.; Dunn, W.B.; Allwood, J.W.; Golovanov, A.P.; Goodacre, R. Fingerprinting food: Current technologies for the detection of food adulteration and contamination. *Chem. Soc. Rev.* **2012**, *41*, 5706–5727. [CrossRef] [PubMed]
51. Elzey, B.; Pollard, D.; Fakayode, S.O. Determination of Adulterated of Neem Oil and Flaxseed Oil Compositions by FTIR Spectroscopy and Multivariate Regression Analysis. *Food Control* **2016**, *68*, 303–309. [CrossRef]
52. Elzey, B.; Norman, V.; Stephenson, J.; Pollard, D.; Fakayode, S.O. Purity Analysis of Adulterated Essential Oils (Wintergreen, Tea Tree, Rosemary, and Lemon Eucalyptus Oil) by FTIR Spectroscopy and Partial-least-square Regression. *Spectroscopy* **2016**, *31*, 26–37.
53. Carrín, M.E.; Carelli, A.A. Peanut oil: Compositional data. *Eur. J. Lipid Sci. Technol.* **2010**, *112*, 697–707. [CrossRef]
54. Dorschel, C. Characterization of the TAG of peanut oil by electrospray LC-MS-MS. *J. Am. Oil Chem. Soc.* **2002**, *79*, 749–753. [CrossRef]
55. List, G.R. Processing and Food Uses of Peanut Oil and Protein. In *Peanut: Genetics, Processing, and Utilization*; Academic Press and AOCS Press: Washington, IL, USA, 2016; pp. 405–428.
56. Lusas, E.W. Food uses of peanut protein. *J. Am. Oil Chem. Soc.* **1979**, *56*, 425–430. [CrossRef] [PubMed]
57. The Statistics Portal. Production Volume of Peanut Oil Worldwide from 2012/13 to 2017/18 (in Million Metric Tons). Available online: https://www.statista.com/statistics/613483/peanut-oil-production-volume-worldwide/ (accessed on 23 May 2018).
58. Malinowski, E.R. *Factor Analysis in Chemistry*; Wiley: New York, NY, USA, 1991.
59. Martens, H.; Naes, T. *Multivariate Calibration*; Wiley: New York, NY, USA, 1998.
60. Adams, M.J. *Chemometrics in Analytical Spectroscopy*, 2nd ed.; Royal Society of Chemistry: Cambridge, MA, USA, 1995.
61. Beebe, K.R.; Pell, R.J.; Seasholtz, M.B. *Chemometrics: A Practical Guide*; John Wiley Publishing: New York, NY, USA, 1998; p. 348.
62. Otto, M. *Pattern Recognition and Classification, in Chemometrics*; John Wiley & Sons Publishing: New York, NY, USA, 2016; pp. 135–211.

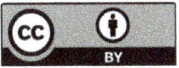

© 2018 by the authors. Licensee MDPI, Basel, Switzerland. This article is an open access article distributed under the terms and conditions of the Creative Commons Attribution (CC BY) license (http://creativecommons.org/licenses/by/4.0/).

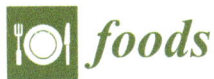

Article

Multistep Optimization of β-Glucosidase Extraction from Germinated Soybeans (*Glycine max* L. Merril) and Recovery of Isoflavone Aglycones

Luciane Yuri Yoshiara [1], Tiago Bervelieri Madeira [2], Adriano Costa de Camargo [1,3,*], Fereidoon Shahidi [3] and Elza Iouko Ida [1]

1. Food Science Department, Londrina State University, Rod. Celso Garcia, KM 380, 86051-990 Londrina, PR, Brazil; lyoshiara@hotmail.com (L.Y.Y.); elida@uel.br (E.I.I.)
2. Chemistry Department, Londrina State University, Rod. Celso Garcia, KM 380, 86051-990 Londrina, PR, Brazil; madeiratb@gmail.com
3. Department of Biochemistry, Memorial University of Newfoundland, St. John's, NL A1B 3X9, Canada; fshahidi@mun.ca
* Correspondence: adrianoesalq@gmail.com; Tel.: +55-19-99876-1128

Received: 21 June 2018; Accepted: 12 July 2018; Published: 13 July 2018

Abstract: Epicotyls from germinated soybeans (EGS) have great potential as sources of endogenous β-glucosidase. Furthermore, this enzyme may improve the conversion of isoflavones into their corresponding aglycones. β-Glucosidase may also increase the release of aglycones from the cell wall of the plant materials. Therefore, the aim of this work was to optimize both the extraction of β-glucosidase from EGS and to further examine its application in defatted soybean cotyledon to improve the recovery of aglycones, which were evaluated by ultra-high performance liquid chromatography (UHPLC). A multistep optimization was carried out and the effects of temperature and pH were investigated by applying a central composite design. The linear effect of pH and the quadratic effect of pH and temperature were significant for the extraction of β-glucosidase and recovery aglycones, respectively. Optimum extraction of β-glucosidase from EGS occurred at 30 °C and pH 5.0. Furthermore, the maximum recovery of aglycones (98.7%), which occurred at 35 °C and pH 7.0–7.6 during 144 h of germination, increased 8.5 times with respect to the lowest concentration. The higher bioaccessibility of aglycones when compared with their conjugated counterparts is well substantiated. Therefore, the data provided in this contribution may be useful for enhancing the benefits of soybean, their products, and/or their processing by-products.

Keywords: endogenous enzyme; phenolic compounds; ultra-high performance liquid chromatography; response surface methodology

1. Introduction

Isoflavones are recognized in human health due to several biological properties, whereas in plants these bioactive compounds also have antifungal properties, thus protecting the plants against plant pathogens [1]. Epidemiological studies have shown that isoflavones may help reduce the risk of some chronic diseases [2]. In humans, a higher incidence of some types of cancers (e.g., breast and colon cancer) and heart disease has been observed in Western populations that consume lower amounts of soy isoflavones compared with the Asian population [3]. According to Brandi [4], isoflavones may reduce bone loss, decrease the risk of development of osteoporosis, and attenuate the symptoms of menopause in women. Because of their structural and molecular weight similarity to the group of female hormones secreted by ovarian cells (estrogens), isoflavones are also known as phytoestrogens [5].

Soybean isoflavones can be found in 12 different forms: β-glycosidics, which have a glucose unit linked to the benzene ring (e.g., daidzin, genistin, and glycitin); β-glycosidic conjugated forms, acetylglycosidics (e.g., acetyldaidzin, acetylgenistin, and acetylglycitin), and malonylglycosidics (e.g., malonyldaidzin, malonylgenistin, and malonylglycitin); and the aglycone forms (e.g., daidzein, genistein, and glycitein), which are not linked to glucose [6]. However, the contribution of the conjugated forms in soybeans are higher compared with that of the aglycone counterparts [7]. Furthermore, soybeans are regarded as the only high-level edible source of isoflavones. The distribution and content of different isoflavones are influenced by multiple factors, such as genetic variety, growth location, and crop year [8]. Likewise, isoflavone contents may vary among different soybean seed components. In fact, only minor amounts of isoflavones are present in the seed coat whereas the hypocotyls contain high concentrations and the cotyledons have been reported to contain 80–90% of the total isoflavones in the seed [9]. However, despite all these variations, the potential health benefits of soybeans as sources of isoflavones are well substantiated.

Walsh et al. [10] conducted an in vitro experiment to screen the stability and bioaccessibility of isoflavones from soy bread. According to these authors, micellarization may be required for optimal bioaccessibility of isoflavones in the aglycone forms. Furthermore, they suggested that the bioavailability of isoflavones from foods containing fat and protein may exceed that from supplements due to enhanced bile secretion. Therefore, due to the high protein content in soybeans, soybean products may be better sources of bioaccessible isoflavones. Isoflavones in the aglycone form are absorbed faster than their conjugated counterparts; therefore, they may render higher biological activities than the latter ones [11,12].

β-glucosidase catalyzes the hydrolysis of conjugated isoflavones, thus generating their respective aglycones. During the hydration of soybeans, this enzyme hydrolyzes glycosidic isoflavones, which affords their respective aglycones [13]. β-Glucosidase (β-D-glucoside glucohydrolase, EC 3.2.1.21), which is commonly found in plants or as part of the metabolism of fungi and bacteria [14], catalyzes the hydrolysis of β-glycosidic di- and/or other glycoside conjugates and oligosaccharides from phenolic compounds, thus releasing both the sugar moiety and the aglycone. Because of this property, a high interest in applying β-glucosidase to increase the amount of aglycone isoflavones in soybean and soy products has been noted [15,16]. In intact plant tissues, β-glucosidases are stored in compartments separated from the substrate, thus playing an important role in the physiology of the plant. During germination, these enzymes act during the process of degradation and lignification of the cell walls of the plant material. Furthermore, they also act as plant growth regulators and during the activation of compounds related to the plant defense [17,18].

The activation of enzymes (e.g., β-glucosidase) occurs during germination [19]. Therefore, germinated soybean components may be a good source of endogenous β-glucosidase which can be extracted and further applied in soy products, thus improving the final products due to higher contents of highly bioaccessible phenolic bioactives [20]. In epicotyls from germinated soybeans (EGS), the specific activity of the crude β-glucosidase extract has been reported to be 72-fold higher than that of the cotyledon extract from ungerminated soybeans and 5.8-fold higher than that of the crude cotyledon extract from germinated soybeans under the same conditions. Therefore, epicotyls have been recommended as a potential industrial source of endogenous β-glucosidase for hydrolysis of conjugated isoflavones to obtain aglycones [21].

The extraction of endogenous β-glucosidases and the use of this enzyme for isoflavone conversion have not yet been well explored in comparison to those of enzymes of microbial origin. Furthermore, the central composite design (CCD) method is an important experimental design used in response surface methodology to construct a second-order model for the response variable without needing a complete three-level factorial experiment, thus reducing the number of experiments while providing trustworthy results. Response surface methodology (RSM) has been successfully used for developing, improving, and optimizing different processes, including the procurement and/or extraction of phenolic compounds [22–24]. Therefore, due to the importance of β-glucosidase, and the existing knowledge gap in the literature, the objective of this work was to use CCD to optimize both the extraction of β-glucosidase from EGS and to establish the best conditions to convert glycosidic isoflavones into their corresponding aglycones by treatment with extracts containing β-glucosidase.

2. Materials and Methods

2.1. Materials

Soybeans (cv. BRS 257) were developed by Embrapa Soybean (Londrina, PR, Brazil). Aglycones (daidzein, glicitein, and genistein) and acetylglucosides standards (daidzin, glycitin, genistin) were purchased from Sigma-Aldrich (Saint Louis, MO, USA). The remaining solvents and chemicals were of analytical or HPLC grade.

2.2. Soybean Germination Process

A previous study was used to select the germination conditions [21]. In this process, 15 germination paper rolls with 50 seeds each were placed in a germination chamber (Marconi, MA 835, Brazil). The seeds were then subjected to a photoperiod of 10 h of light per day. The temperature was kept at 35 °C (±1 °C) and controlled relative humidity (100%) for 144 h [21]. The epicotyls were manually separated, freeze-dried (Christ, ALPHA 1-4 LD plus, Germany), ground (A11 Basic Mill, Ika, Brazil), and stored at −26 °C until analysis.

2.3. CCD-Based Optimization of Extraction of Active β-Glucosidase

The effect of temperature (X_1 = 23, 25, 30, 35, and 37 °C) and pH (X_2 = 3.6, 4.0, 5.0, 6.0, and 6.4) on the extraction of active β-glucosidase from EGS was evaluated by applying the CCD with 5 levels of variation in a total of 11 assays (Table 1). Therefore, the response function (Y) stems from the β-glucosidase activity. The extraction procedure was performed as described by Carrão-Panizzi and Bordingnon [25] using 0.1 mol L^{-1} sodium citrate buffer with 0.1 mol L^{-1} NaCl at various pH values (X_1) and temperatures (X_2), according to the experimental design. The extraction procedure (100 mg of EGS in 1.5 mL sodium citrate buffer) was conducted under agitation for 50 min. After centrifugation at 2500× g (Cientec, CT 600, Piracicaba, Brazil) for 15 min, the extract so obtained was used for determination of β-glucosidase activity.

Table 1. Independent variables and variation levels for the central composite design for optimization of the extraction of active β-glucosidase from epicotyls from geminated soybeans.

Independent Variables	Variation Levels				
	−1.41	−1	0	+1	+1.41
X_1 = Temperature (°C)	23	25	30	35	37
X_2 = pH	3.6	4.0	5.0	6.0	6.4

2.4. CCD-Based Optimization of β-Glucosidase-Assisted Conversion of Conjugated Isoflavones into Their Corresponding Aglycones

Extracts with the highest β-glucosidase activity were used in this step of the experiment. A CCD with 2 variables (X_3 = temperature and X_4 = pH) and 5 variation levels (Table 2) in 2 blocks was used. The first block consisted of a 2^2 factorial design, a total of 7 assays (assays 1–7), and 2 variables with 3 variation levels (X_3 = 20, 35, and 50 °C and X_4 = pH 4.0, 5.5, and 7.0). The second block, with a total of 6 assays (assays 8–13) containing the axial points of the CCD (X_3 = 13.9 and 56.2 °C and X_4 = pH 3.39, and 7.61), was performed to verify the quadratic effects. Previous experiments were conducted (data not shown) and the maximum conversion was achieved at 14 h of hydrolysis. The assays were performed randomly with defatted soybean cotyledon flours in 3.0 mL buffer (1:10 w/v). According to each design, the pH values were adjusted with 0.1 M sodium phosphate and 0.1 M citric acid solutions. To each test tube, 5.0 units of β-glucosidase activity from EGS were added and shaken for 14 h at temperatures described in Table 2. The samples were freeze-dried and used for identification and quantification of isoflavones by ultra-high performance liquid chromatography (UHPLC). The response function stems from the percentage of aglycones (W = % aglycones) obtained in relation to the total isoflavone content present in each sample.

Table 2. Independent variables and variation levels for the central composite design for optimization of the conversion of conjugated isoflavones into their corresponding aglycones.

Independent Variables	Variation Levels				
	−1.41	−1	0	+1	+1.41
X_3 = Temperature (°C)	13.9	20.0	35.0	50.0	56.2
X_4 = pH	3.39	4.00	5.50	7.00	7.61

2.5. Determination of β-Glucosidase Activity

The enzymatic activity was determined according to the method described in the literature [26] with slight modifications. Briefly, 0.4 mL of 16 mM *p*-nitrophenyl-beta-D-glucopyranoside and 0.1 M phosphate–citrate buffer (pH 5.0) were transferred to a test tube and placed in a water bath at 30 °C for 10 min. The sample (0.1 mL) was added and the test tubes were placed in a water bath at 30 °C for 30 min more. The reaction was terminated with the addition of 0.5 M sodium carbonate (0.5 mL). The concentration of *p*-nitrophenol released during the reaction was determined by reading the absorbance at 420 nm with a spectrophotometer (Biochrom Libra S22, Cambridge, England). For quantification, a *p*-nitrophenol (20–160 mM) calibration curve was prepared. One unit of enzyme activity (UA) was defined as the amount of β-glucosidase that releases 1 mM *p*-nitrophenol min^{-1}. The results were expressed as units of β-glucosidase activity (UA mL^{-1}) per milliliter of extract.

2.6. Extraction and Determination of Isoflavones by Ultra-High-Performance Liquid Chromatography (UHPLC)

Defatted cotyledon soy flours subjected to enzymatic conversion were used for extraction. Water/ethanol/acetone (1:1:1 $v/v/v$) was used for the extraction of isoflavones. The samples (250 mg) were mixed with 6 mL of solvent and the extraction was performed under sonication at 60 °C for 10 min [27]. After centrifugation and filtration (Millex–LH filters; 0.20 µm) of the supernatant, the extracts (1.4 µL) were injected into the UHPLC (Acquity UPLC®System), with automatic system injection, oven with controlled temperature at 35 °C, and a diode array detector (Waters, Milford, MA, USA). A reversed-phase column, BEH C18 (Waters, 2.1 mm × 50 mm, 1.7 µm particles), was used. The binary mobile phase consisted of acidified water (glacial acetic acid, pH 3.0)—mobile phase A—and acetonitrile—mobile phase B. The elution gradient used was as follows: 0 min, 90% A and 10% B; 8 min, 0% A and 100% B. The initial condition was re-established at 9 min. The total run took 12 min and the flow rate was 0.70 mL min^{-1}. The temperature was kept constant (35 °C) and a diode array detector (Waters) with a wavelength set at 260 nm was used. Isoflavones, namely daidzin, glycitin, genistin, daidzein, glicitein, and genistein, were identified and quantified by comparing their retention times and UV spectra with coded and authentic standards under the same conditions as the samples. The presence of acetyldaidzin, acetylgenistin, and acetylglycitin was also investigated with coded and authentic standards. However, they were not detected in any of the samples tested and/or treatments; this is common for raw soybeans [6]. According to the literature [28], malonylglucosides (malonyldaidzin, malonylglycitin, and malonylgenistin) were quantified based on the standard curves of the corresponding β-glycosidic isoflavones (daidzin, glycitin, and genistin, respectively) using the similarity of the extinction coefficients. Limits of detection and quantification for listed compounds ranged from 0.003 to 0.0239 and from 0.009 to 0.725 µg/mL, respectively. Regression coefficients of the plotted graphs had R^2 ranging from 0.9988 to 0.9996.

2.7. Statistical Analysis

STATISTICA 8.0 software (StatSoft, Palo Alto, CA, USA) was used to determine the effects of independent variables, calculate the regression coefficient (R^2), perform analysis of variance (ANOVA), and build the response surfaces at 5% significance. Data were adjusted to a second-order polynomial model (Equation (1)):

$$y = \beta_0 + \beta_1 x_1 + \beta_2 x_2 + \beta_{11} x_1^2 + \beta_{22} x_2^2 + \beta_{12} x_1 x_2 \quad (1)$$

where y is the response variable; x_1 and x_2 are the coded process variables; and β_0, β_1, β_2, β_{11}, β_{22}, and β_{12} are the regression coefficients.

To evaluate and validate the mathematical models, a new assay was performed under the conditions (X_1 = °C and X_2 = pH) that yielded the extracts with higher activity of β-glucosidase from EGS and the highest conversion of conjugated isoflavones into their respective aglycones (X_3 = °C and X_4 = pH). The observed model was obtained under experimental conditions, and the calculated values ($\hat{y}$ and $\hat{w}$) were determined using the proposed model. The model was validated and the observed responses were within the confidence interval of the model.

3. Results and Discussion

3.1. Optimization of β-Glucosidase Extraction from Germinated Soybean Epicotyls

The linear effect of the variable X_1 (temperature) on the response function y (β-glucosidase activity) was not significant, whereas the linear effect of the variable X_2 (pH) was significant. In contrast, the quadratic effects of the variables X_1 and X_2 were significant but the interaction between the variables X_1 and X_2 was not significant (Table 3). These results indicated that variable X_2 (pH between 3.6 and 6.4) was essential to obtaining extracts with high β-glucosidase activity from epicotyls from germinated soybeans.

Table 3. Analysis of variance (ANOVA) for the β-glucosidase activity of extracts obtained from epicotyls from germinated soybeans.

Variation Source	SS	DF	MS	F Test	p	R^2
X_1 (T) (linear)	0.558	1	0.558	0.659	0.428	0.94
X_1 (T) (quadratic)	19.038	1	19.038	22.492	0.002	
X_2 (pH) (linear)	62.340	1	62.340	73.650	0.000	
X_2 (pH) (quadratic)	137.038	1	137.038	161.900	0.000	
Interaction $X_1 X_2$	0.120	1	0.120	0.142	0.711	
Error	13.543	16	0.846			
Total	214.527	21				

SS = sum square. DF = degrees of freedom. MS = mean square. T = temperature in °C.

The determination coefficient (R^2) of 0.94 indicates that 94% of the experimental data fitted the model. The polynomial model (Y) representing the activity of β-glucosidase of extracts from EGS is described below:

$$Y = 11.39 + 0.18 x_1 - 1.29 x_1^2 - 1.97 x_2 - 3.48 x_2^2 + 0.12 x_1 x_2 \quad (2)$$

where x_1 and x_2 are the coded variables representing the temperature and pH, respectively, for the optimum recovery of high-activity β-glucosidase extracts from EGS.

According to the results in Table 4, extracts obtained at 30 or 35 °C and low pH values of 3.6 or 4.0 (assays 10 and 3, respectively) showed lower β-glucosidase activity. In contrast, higher β-glucosidase activity was found in extracts obtained at 23 °C and pH 5.0 (assay 8), 25 °C and pH 6.0 (assay 2), 30 °C and pH 6.4 (assay 11), and 37 °C and pH 5.0 (assay 9). Finally, the response surface (Figure 1) shows that the highest β-glucosidase activity was obtained when the extractions were performed at the central point, i.e., at 30 °C and pH 5.0 (assays 5, 6, and 7). Furthermore, extracts with high β-glucosidase activity could also be obtained at temperatures ranging from 27.5 to 33.5 °C and pH from 4.9 to 5.5. The conditions used as the central point were also in good agreement with the desirability parameter of the proposed model (Figure 2), thus supporting the procurement of extracts with a high β-glucosidase activity at 30 °C and pH 5.0.

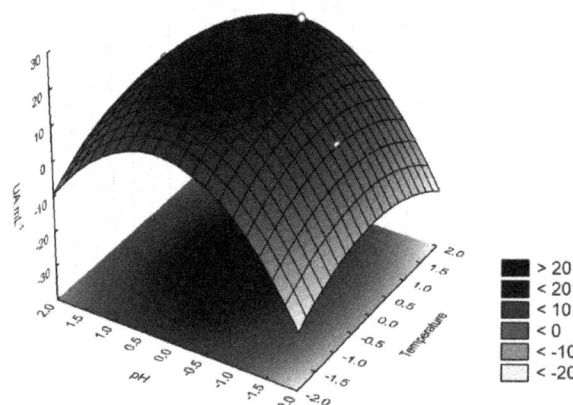

Figure 1. Surface response for the activity of β-glucosidase (UA mL^{-1}) from epicotyls from germinated soybeans.

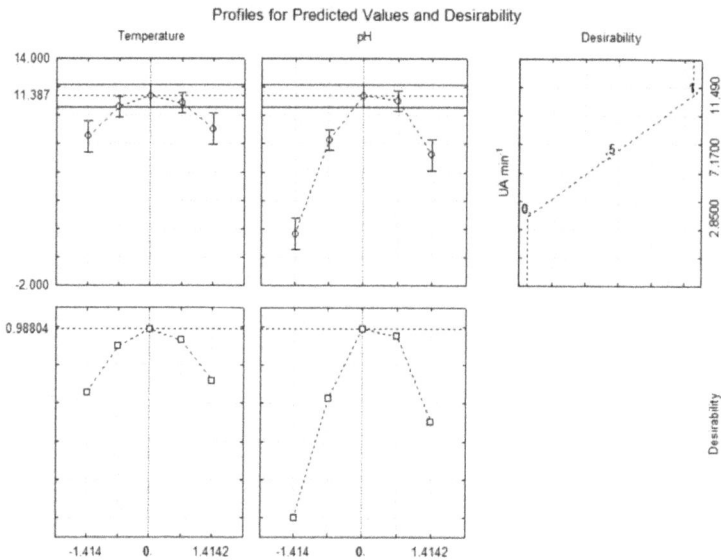

Figure 2. Profiles for predicted values and desirability for β-glucosidase activity of extracts from epicotyls from germinated soybeans.

Table 4. Central composite design with two coded (x_1 and x_2) and decoded (X_1 and X_2) variables and the response function (Y) for the activity of β-glucosidase from epicotyls from germinated soybeans.

Assays	Coded Variables		Decoded Variable		Response Function (Y)
	x_1	x_2	T (°C) (X_1)	pH (X_2)	β-Glucosidase Activity (UA mL^{-1})
1	−1	−1	25.0	4.0	8.16
2	−1	1	25.0	6.0	17.7
3	1	−1	35.0	4.0	6.22
4	1	1	35.0	6.0	16.7
5	0	0	30.0	5.0	22.4
6	0	0	30.0	5.0	23.0
7	0	0	30.0	5.0	23.0
8	−1.41	0	23.0	5.0	16.5
9	1.41	0	37.0	5.0	20.7
10	0	−1.41	30.0	3.6	5.76
11	0	1.41	30.0	6.4	13.9

Matsuura and Obata [26] extracted, partially purified, and characterized β-glucosidases from soybean cotyledons under different conditions including lower temperatures (between −10 and 5 °C). Although the extraction of β-glucosidase from cotyledons has been studied by these authors, to the best of our knowledge, the procurement of extracts with high β-glucosidase activity from germinated soybean epicotyls has not been reported in the literature. Furthermore, our proposed model proved to be advantageous to establish the best conditions to obtain extracts with high enzyme activity. In addition, working at 30 °C offers more operational advantages compared to the lower temperatures (between −10 and 5 °C) reported in the literature [26]. The proposed model was validated with an additional experiment under optimal conditions and the results (Figure 4) fell within the confidence interval of the estimated response, thus confirming the validity of the model.

3.2. Optimization of the Recovery of Aglycones Using β-Glucosidase from Germinated Soybean Epicotyls

According to variance analysis (ANOVA), the linear effect of the variable X_4 (pH) and quadratic effects of the variables X_3 (°C) and X_4 (pH) were significant. However, the effects of the block, linear variable X_3 (°C), and the interaction of the variables X_3 (°C) and X_4 (pH) on the response (W = % aglycones) were not significant (Table 5). Therefore, nonsignificant terms were excluded from the model which did not affect the R^2. The coefficient of determination (R^2) was 0.86, in other words, 86% of experimental data can be explained by the model. Therefore, Equation (3) is described as follows:

$$W = 81.938 + 22.328x_4 - 11.231x_4^2 - 13.8562x_3^2 \tag{3}$$

where W = % aglycones and x_3 and x_4 are the coded variables representing the temperature and pH, respectively.

Table 5. Analysis of variance (ANOVA) for the conversion of conjugated isoflavones into their corresponding aglycones.

Variation Source	SS	DF	MS	F test	p	R^2
Block	22.050	1	22.050	0.17864	0.683680	0.86
(X_4) pH (Linear)	4217.201	1	4217.201	34.16513	0.000385	
(X_4) pH (Quadratic)	872.759	1	872.759	7.07055	0.028848	
(X_3) T (Quadratic)	1328.402	1	1328.402	10.76189	0.011179	
Error	987.486	8	123.436			
Total	7231.600	12				

SS = sum square. DF = degrees of freedom. MS = mean square. T = temperature in °C.

The aglycone content of the soybean cotyledon flour (BRS 257) devoid of β-glucosidase addition was 2.9% and, regardless of the temperature (X_3), reached values higher than 47% (Table 6) with greater pH (X_4) values (0, +1, and +1.41). This suggests a greater pH influence on the response function (W = % of aglycones), thus supporting the screening of the main effects.

Table 6. Central composite design with two coded (x_3 and x_4) and decoded (X_3 and X_4) variables and the response function (W) for the conversion of conjugated isoflavones into their corresponding aglycones.

Assays	Block	Coded Variables		Decoded Variables		Response Function (W)
		x_3	x_4	T (°C) (X_3)	pH (X_4)	% Aglycones *
1	1	−1	−1	20.0	4.00	47.5
2	1	+1	−1	50.0	4.00	44.6
3	1	−1	+1	20.0	7.00	68.6
4	1	+1	+1	50.0	7.00	84.0
5 (c)	1	0	0	35.0	5.50	88.6
6 (c)	1	0	0	35.0	5.50	79.0
7 (c)	1	0	0	35.0	5.50	88.6
8	2	0	−1.41	35.0	3.39	11.6
9	2	0	+1.41	35.0	7.61	98.7
10	2	−1.41	0	13.9	5.50	48.6
11	2	+1.41	0	56.2	5.50	47.1
12 (c)	2	0	0	35.0	5.50	85.0
13 (c)	2	0	0	35.0	5.50	88.3

* % aglycone isoflavones relative to total isoflavones extracted, determined by ultra-high-performance liquid chromatography (UHPLC). High-aglycone defatted soybean cotyledon flours were produced by treatment with β-glucosidase from germinated soybean epicotyls. "c" is central point.

The response surface (Figure 3) shows a region at which more than 80% of the isoflavones recovered were in the aglycone form, i.e., a pH range between +0.5 and +1.5 (6.25 < pH < 7.75) and a temperature between −0.5 and +0.5 (27.5 < T < 42.5). Furthermore, an optimum region at which the maximum percentage of isoflavones in the aglycone form was recovered could be determined. The desirability parameter indicates two optimal points of maximum (W = 98.7% aglycones), i.e., when x_3 = 0 (35 °C) and x_4 = +1 or +1.41 (pH = 7.00 and 7.61). One of these test points coincides with assay 9 (Z = 98.7% aglycones). These results are distinct from the optimum conditions of pH (between 5.2 and 6.0) and temperature (50 °C) for β-glucosidase activity from soybean cell tissue described by Hosel and Todenhagen [29] and by Matsuura and Obata [30] who reported optimal activity at pH 4.5 and a temperature of 45 °C for a soybean β-glucosidase. However, the proposed models were validated for both response functions which were within the confidence interval of the model (Figure 4).

A complete conversion of glycosidic isoflavones into their aglycones has been described by other authors [31]. However, their study was conducted with β-glucosidase from microbial origin (*Lactobacillus* (L.) *rhamnosus* CRL981). Furthermore, Song and Yu [32] applied β-glucosidase from *Thermotoga maritima* to recombinant soybean flour and obtained an almost complete conversion of all isoflavone glycosides. Endogenous β-glucosidases represent a more secure source of β-glucosidases than microbial sources. However, endogenous β-glucosidases have been poorly explored when compared with the microbial conversion of conjugated isoflavones into their aglycone forms. As mentioned before, in the present study, the maximum aglycone isoflavones obtained was 98.7% when endogenous β-glucosidase from EGS was used under the two conditions described above, therefore providing strong evidence on the potential use of EGS as a great source of endogenous β-glucosidase.

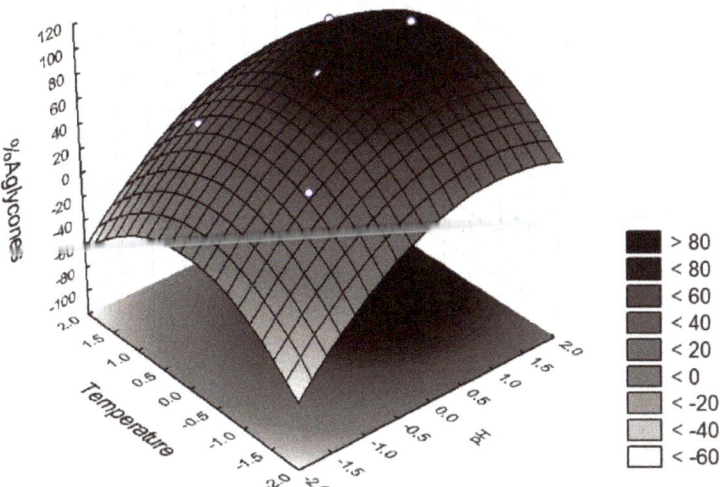

Figure 3. Surface response for the conversion of glycosidic isoflavones into their corresponding aglycones. High-aglycone defatted soybean cotyledon flours were produced by treatment with β-glucosidase from germinated soybean epicotyls.

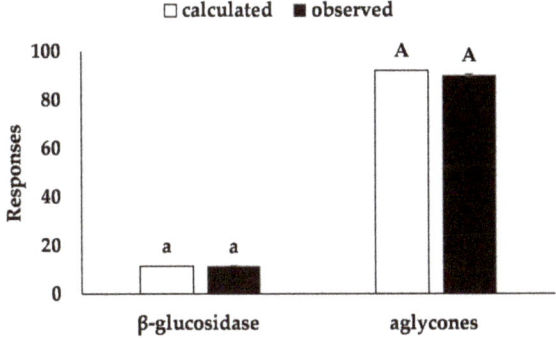

Figure 4. Validation of the models proposed for the procurement of extracts with β-glucosidase from epicotyls from germinated soybeans and high-aglycone defatted soybean cotyledon flours. Means with the same lower case (β-glucosidase) or capital (aglycones) letters: results fall within the confidence interval of the generated model.

Several pieces of evidence have demonstrated that different plant parts may present different phenolic compounds [33–39], therefore suggesting that the expression of genes associated with the production of some enzymes may be tissue specific. Likewise, not only the absorption of the phenolics is important but also their structure/activity [40–42]. Perera et al. [40] demonstrated that epigallocatechin gallate derivatives procured via lipophilization showed enhanced antioxidant properties compared with those of epigallocatechin gallate. Likewise, Oh and Shahidi [42] reported that several lipophilized resveratrol derivatives had better hydrogen peroxide scavenging activity than resveratrol. In addition, Oldoni et al. [41] demonstrated that minor changes such as the position of the hydroxyl group in flavonoids may be responsible for major changes in their final effects. According to their study, the concentration of procyanidin A2 necessary to scavenge 50% of the DPPH radical was 1.7-fold higher than that of procyanidin A1. Besides the antioxidant activity, which may be related to the inhibition of low-density lipoprotein cholesterol oxidation and DNA damage [43,44], phenolic compounds have been regarded as potential inhibitors of enzymes related to the absorption of carbohydrates and lipids [38,45]. In a bioactivity-guided isolation and purification study to identify α-glucosidase inhibitors, Sun et al. [46] suggested that C_1-OH of the saccharide moiety in phenolic glycosides are necessary for a potent inhibition of intestinal α-glucosidases. According to Bustanji et al. [47], the inhibitory effect towards lipase activity was in the order of gallic acid > caffeic acid > chlorogenic acid > rosmarinic acid. A recent study [37] also demonstrated that whereas proanthocyanidin-rich extracts showed higher antioxidant activity, the extracts containing only phenolic acids showed higher antimicrobial effects. Finally, inflammation has been linked to several health issues, including those related to oxidative stress. A myriad of phenolic compounds have been reported to act as potential anti-inflammatory and antioxidant compounds [39,48–50] and the link between inflammatory responses and several diseases is well recognized. According to Lee et al. [51], fermented soymilk with greater contents of isoflavones in the aglycone form also showed higher antioxidant properties. The importance of natural product characterization in studies related to their bioactivity has long been discussed [52,53]. Therefore, by understanding the best conditions to produce β-glucosidase from EGS as well as its further application in the procurement of high-aglycone defatted soybean cotyledon flours, the present study contributes to both basic and applied science related to food bioactives and health.

4. Conclusions

EGS was demonstrated to be of great potential as a source of endogenous β-glucosidase. Furthermore, two models were optimized, both for the extraction of β-glucosidase from EGS and for further application in defatted soybean cotyledon flour. Optimum extraction of β-glucosidase from EGS was procured at 30 °C and pH 5.0 whereas the maximum recovery of aglycones (98.7%) occurred at 35 °C and pH ranging from 7.0 to 7.6. The higher bioaccessibility of aglycones when compared with their conjugated counterparts has already been discussed by other authors [54,55]. Furthermore, the structure/activity has also been in the spotlight. Therefore, by reporting the best conditions to obtain a high-aglycone soybean feedstock, the present contribution may be useful for enhancing knowledge about the potential benefits of soybean products and/or processing by-products.

Author Contributions: Conceptualization, E.I.I. and L.Y.Y.; Methodology, A.C.d.C., E.I.I., L.Y.Y.; Software, L.Y.Y. and T.B.M.; Validation, L.Y.Y. and T.B.M.; Formal Analysis, L.Y.Y. and T.B.M.; Investigation, L.Y.Y. and T.B.M.; Resources, E.I.I.; Data Curation, L.Y.Y.; Writing—Original Draft Preparation, E.I.I. and L.Y.Y.; Writing—Review & Editing, A.C.d.C., E.I.I., F.S., and L.Y.Y.; Supervision, E.I.I.; Project Administration, E.I.I.; Funding Acquisition, E.I.I.

Funding: This research was partially funded by CNPq/MCT and Fundação Araucária/PR. L. Y. Yoshiara and T. B. Madeira would like to thank CNPq for their PhD and undergraduate scholarships, respectively. F. Shahidi thanks the Natural Science and Engineering Research Council (NSERC) of Canada for partial financial support. A. C. de Camargo is thankful to Coordination of Improvement of Higher Education–Ministry of Education of Brazil–CAPES for his postdoctoral fellowship. E. I. Ida is a CNPq Research Fellow.

Acknowledgments: The authors are thankful to Embrapa Soybean (Londrina, PR, Brazil) for providing the soybeans used in this investigation.

Conflicts of Interest: The authors declare no conflict of interest.

References

1. Hsieh, M.-C.; Graham, T.L. Partial purification and characterization of a soybean β-glucosidase with high specific activity towards isoflavone conjugates. *Phytochemistry* **2001**, *58*, 995–1005. [CrossRef]

2. Villares, A.; Rostagno, M.A.; García-Lafuente, A.; Guillamón, E.; Martínez, J.A. Content and profile of isoflavones in soy-based foods as a function of the production process. *Food Bioprocess Technol.* **2011**, *4*, 27–38. [CrossRef]
3. He, F.-J.; Chen, J.-Q. Consumption of soybean, soy foods, soy isoflavones and breast cancer incidence: Differences between Chinese women and women in western countries and possible mechanisms. *Food Sci. Hum. Wellness* **2013**, *2*, 146–161. [CrossRef]
4. Brandi, M.L. Natural and synthetic isoflavones in the prevention and treatment of chronic diseases. *Calcif. Tissue Int.* **1997**, *61*, S5–S8. [CrossRef] [PubMed]
5. Adlercreutz, H.; Mazur, W. Phyto-oestrogens and western diseases. *Ann. Med.* **1997**, *29*, 95–120. [CrossRef] [PubMed]
6. Falcão, H.G.; Handa, C.L.; Silva, M.B.R.; de Camargo, A.C.; Shahidi, F.; Kurozawa, L.E.; Ida, E.I. Soybean ultrasound pre-treatment prior to soaking affects β-glucosidase activity, isoflavone profile and soaking time. *Food Chem.* **2018**. [CrossRef]
7. Kudou, S.; Fleury, Y.; Welti, D.; Magnolato, D.; Uchida, T.; Kitamura, K.; Okubo, K. Malonyl isoflavone glycosides in soybean seeds (*Glycine max* Merrill). *Agric. Biol. Chem.* **1991**, *55*, 2227–2233. [CrossRef]
8. Wang, H.J.; Murphy, P.A. Isoflavone content in commercial soybean foods. *J. Agric. Food Chem.* **1994**, *42*, 1666–1673. [CrossRef]
9. Tsukamoto, C.; Shimada, S.; Igita, K.; Kudou, S.; Kokubun, M.; Okubo, K.; Kitamura, K. Factors affecting isoflavone content in soybean seeds: Changes in isoflavones, saponins, and composition of fatty acids at different temperatures during seed development. *J. Agric. Food Chem.* **1995**, *43*, 1184–1192. [CrossRef]
10. Walsh, K.R.; Zhang, Y.C.; Vodovotz, Y.; Schwartz, S.J.; Failla, M.L. Stability and bioaccessibility of isoflavones from soy bread during in vitro digestion. *J. Agric. Food Chem.* **2003**, *51*, 4603–4609. [CrossRef] [PubMed]
11. Fukutake, M.; Takahashi, M.; Ishida, K.; Kawamura, H.; Sugimura, T.; Wakabayashi, K. Quantification of genistein and genistin in soybeans and soybean products. *Food Chem. Toxicol.* **1996**, *34*, 457–461. [CrossRef]
12. Izumi, T.; Piskula, M.K.; Osawa, S.; Obata, A.; Tobe, K.; Saito, M.; Kataoka, S.; Kubota, Y.; Kikuchi, M. Soy isoflavone aglycones are absorbed faster and in higher amounts than their glucosides in humans. *J. Nutr.* **2000**, *130*, 1695–1699. [CrossRef] [PubMed]
13. Matsuura, M.; Obata, A.; Fukushima, D. Objectionable flavor of soy milk developed during the soaking of soybeans and its control. *J. Food Sci.* **1989**, *54*, 602–605. [CrossRef]
14. Esen, A. Purification and partial characterization of maize (*Zea mays* L.) beta-glucosidase. *Plant Physiol.* **1992**, *98*, 174–182. [CrossRef] [PubMed]
15. Kuo, L.C.; Cheng, W.Y.; Wu, R.Y.; Huang, C.J.; Lee, K.T. Hydrolysis of black soybean isoflavone glycosides by *Bacillus subtilis* natto. *Appl. Microbiol. Biotechnol.* **2006**, *73*, 314–320. [CrossRef] [PubMed]
16. Chuankhayan, P.; Rimlumduan, T.; Svasti, J.; Cairns, J.R.K. Hydrolysis of soybean isoflavonoid glycosides by *Dalbergia* β-glucosidases. *J. Agric. Food Chem.* **2007**, *55*, 2407–2412. [CrossRef] [PubMed]
17. Handa, C.L.; Couto, U.R.; Vicensoti, A.H.; Georgetti, S.R.; Ida, E.I. Optimisation of soy flour fermentation parameters to produce β-glucosidase for bioconversion into aglycones. *Food Chem.* **2014**, *152*, 56–65. [CrossRef] [PubMed]
18. Morant, A.V.; Jørgensen, K.; Jørgensen, C.; Paquette, S.M.; Sánchez-Pérez, R.; Møller, B.L.; Bak, S. β-Glucosidases as detonators of plant chemical defense. *Phytochemistry* **2008**, *69*, 1795–1813. [CrossRef] [PubMed]
19. Santosh, T.R.; Balasubramanian, K.K.; Lalitha, K. Enhancement of β-Glucosidase and β-Galactosidase of *Trigonella foenum-graecum* by exposure to the allelochemical mimosine. *J. Agric. Food Chem.* **1999**, *47*, 462–467. [CrossRef] [PubMed]
20. Ribeiro, M.L.L.; Mandarino, J.M.G.; Carrão-Panizzi, M.C.; Oliveira, M.C.N.; Campo, C.B.H.; Nepomuceno, A.L.; Ida, E.I. β-Glucosidase activity and isoflavone content in germinated soybean radicles and cotyledons. *J. Food Biochem.* **2006**, *30*, 453–465. [CrossRef]
21. Yoshiara, L.Y.; Madeira, T.B.; Ribeiro, M.L.L.; Mandarino, J.M.G.; Carrão-Panizzi, M.C.; Ida, E.I. β-Glucosidase activity of soybean (*Glycine max*) embryonic axis germinated in the presence or absence of light. *J. Food Biochem.* **2011**, *36*, 699–705. [CrossRef]
22. Ferreres, F.; Grosso, C.; Gil-Izquierdo, A.; Valentão, P.; Mota, A.T.; Andrade, P.B. Optimization of the recovery of high-value compounds from pitaya fruit by-products using microwave-assisted extraction. *Food Chem.* **2017**, *230*, 463–474. [CrossRef] [PubMed]

23. He, B.; Zhang, L.-L.; Yue, X.-Y.; Liang, J.; Jiang, J.; Gao, X.-L.; Yue, P.-X. Optimization of ultrasound-assisted extraction of phenolic compounds and anthocyanins from blueberry (*Vaccinium ashei*) wine pomace. *Food Chem.* **2016**, *204*, 70–76. [CrossRef] [PubMed]
24. Liyana-Pathirana, C.; Shahidi, F. Optimization of extraction of phenolic compounds from wheat using response surface methodology. *Food Chem.* **2005**, *93*, 47–56. [CrossRef]
25. Carrão-Panizzi, M.C.; Bordingnon, J.R. Activity of beta-glucosidase and levels of isoflavone glucosides in soybean cultivars affected by the environment. *Pesq. Agropec. Bras.* **2000**, *35*, 873–878. [CrossRef]
26. Matsuura, M.; Sasaki, J.; Murao, S. Studies on β-glucosidases from soybeans that hydrolyze daidzin and genistin: Isolation and characterization of an isozyme. *Biosci. Biotechnol. Biochem.* **1995**, *59*, 1623–1627. [CrossRef]
27. Yoshiara, L.Y.; Madeira, T.B.; Delaroza, F.; Da Silva, J.B.; Ida, E.I. Optimization of soy isoflavone extraction with different solvents using the simplex-centroid mixture design. *Int. J. Food Sci. Nutr.* **2012**, *63*, 978–986. [CrossRef] [PubMed]
28. Coward, L.; Smith, M.; Kirk, M.; Barnes, S. Chemical modification of isoflavones in soyfoods during cooking and processing. *Am. J. Clin. Nutr.* **1998**, *68*, 1486S–1491S. [CrossRef] [PubMed]
29. Hösel, W.; Todenhagen, R. Characterization of a β-glucosidase from *Glycine Max* which hydrolyses coniferin and syringin. *Phytochemistry* **1980**, *19*, 1349–1353. [CrossRef]
30. Matsuura, M.; Obata, A. β-Glucosidases from soybeans hydrolyze daidzin and genistin. *J. Food Sci.* **1993**, *58*, 144–147. [CrossRef]
31. Marazza, J.A.; Garro, M.S.; Savoy de Giori, G. Aglycone production by *Lactobacillus rhamnosus* CRL981 during soymilk fermentation. *Food Microbiol.* **2009**, *26*, 333–339. [CrossRef] [PubMed]
32. Xue, Y.; Song, X.; Yu, J. Overexpression of β-glucosidase from *Thermotoga maritima* for the production of highly purified aglycone isoflavones from soy flour. *World J. Microbiol. Biotechnol.* **2009**, *25*, 2165–2172. [CrossRef]
33. John, J.A.; Shahidi, F. Phenolic compounds and antioxidant activity of Brazil nut (*Bertholletia excelsa*). *J. Funct. Foods* **2010**, *2*, 196–209. [CrossRef]
34. Peng, H.; Li, W.; Li, H.; Deng, Z.; Zhang, B. Extractable and non-extractable bound phenolic compositions and their antioxidant properties in seed coat and cotyledon of black soybean (*Glycinemax* (L.) Merr). *J. Funct. Foods* **2017**, *32*, 296–312. [CrossRef]
35. Arruda, H.S.; Pereira, G.A.; de Morais, D.R.; Eberlin, M.N.; Pastore, G.M. Determination of free, esterified, glycosylated and insoluble-bound phenolics composition in the edible part of araticum fruit (*Annona crassiflora* mart.) and its by-products by HPLC-ESI-MS/MSms. *Food Chem.* **2018**, *245*, 738–749. [CrossRef] [PubMed]
36. Ambigaipalan, P.; de Camargo, A.C.; Shahidi, F. Identification of phenolic antioxidants and bioactives of pomegranate seeds following juice extraction using HPLC-DAD-ESI-MS[n]. *Food Chem.* **2017**, *221*, 1883–1894. [CrossRef] [PubMed]
37. De Camargo, A.C.; Regitano-d'Arce, M.A.B.; Rasera, G.B.; Canniatti-Brazaca, S.G.; do Prado-Silva, L.; Alvarenga, V.O.; Sant'Ana, A.S.; Shahidi, F. Phenolic acids and flavonoids of peanut by-products: Antioxidant capacity and antimicrobial effects. *Food Chem.* **2017**, *237*, 538–544. [CrossRef] [PubMed]
38. De Camargo, A.C.; Regitano-d'Arce, M.A.B.; Shahidi, F. Phenolic profile of peanut by-products: antioxidant potential and inhibition of alpha-glucosidase and lipase activities. *J. Am. Oil Chem. Soc.* **2017**, *94*, 959–971. [CrossRef]
39. Tremocoldi, M.A.; Rosalen, P.L.; Franchin, M.; Massarioli, A.P.; Denny, C.; Daiuto, É.R.; Paschoal, J.A.R.; Melo, P.S.; De Alencar, S.M. Exploration of avocado by-products as natural sources of bioactive compounds. *PLoS ONE* **2018**, *13*, e0192577. [CrossRef] [PubMed]
40. Perera, N.; Ambigaipalan, P.; Shahidi, F. Epigallocatechin gallate (EGCG) esters with different chain lengths fatty acids and their antioxidant activity in food and biological systems. *J. Food Bioact.* **2018**, *1*, 124–133.
41. Oldoni, T.L.C.; Melo, P.S.; Massarioli, A.P.; Moreno, I.A.M.; Bezerra, R.M.N.; Rosalen, P.L.; da Silva, G.V.J.; Nascimento, A.M.; Alencar, S.M. Bioassay-guided isolation of proanthocyanidins with antioxidant activity from peanut (*Arachis hypogaea*) skin by combination of chromatography techniques. *Food Chem.* **2016**, *192*, 306–312. [CrossRef] [PubMed]
42. Oh, W.Y.; Shahidi, F. Antioxidant activity of resveratrol ester derivatives in food and biological model systems. *Food Chem.* **2018**, *261*, 267–273. [CrossRef] [PubMed]

43. Amarowicz, R.; Pegg, R.B. The potential protective effects of phenolic compounds against low-density lipoprotein oxidation. *Curr. Pharm. Des.* **2017**, *23*, 2754–2766. [CrossRef] [PubMed]
44. De Camargo, A.C.; Regitano-d'Arce, M.A.B.; Gallo, C.R.; Shahidi, F. Gamma-irradiation induced changes in microbiological status, phenolic profile and antioxidant activity of peanut skin. *J. Funct. Foods* **2015**, *12*, 129–143. [CrossRef]
45. Rahman, M.J.; de Camargo, A.C.; Shahidi, F. Phenolic and polyphenolic profiles of chia seeds and their in vitro biological activities. *J. Funct. Foods* **2017**, *35*, 622–634. [CrossRef]
46. Sun, S.; Kadouh, H.C.; Zhu, W.; Zhou, K. Bioactivity-guided isolation and purification of α-glucosidase inhibitor, 6-O-D-glycosides, from tinta cão grape pomace. *J. Funct. Foods* **2016**, *23*, 573–579. [CrossRef]
47. Bustanji, Y.; Issa, A.; Mohammad, M.; Hudaib, M.; Tawah, K.; Alkhatib, H.; Almasri, I.; Al-Khalidi, B. Inhibition of hormone sensitive lipase and pancreatic lipase by *Rosmarinus officinalis* extract and selected phenolic constituents. *J. Med. Plant Res.* **2010**, *4*, 2235–2242.
48. Denny, C.; Melo, P.S.; Franchin, M.; Massarioli, A.P.; Bergamaschi, K.B.; De Alencar, S.M.; Rosalen, P.L. Guava pomace: A new source of anti-inflammatory and analgesic bioactives. *BMC Complement. Altern. Med.* **2013**, *13*, 235. [CrossRef] [PubMed]
49. Zhang, H.; Tsao, R. Dietary polyphenols, oxidative stress and antioxidant and anti-inflammatory effects. *Curr. Opin. Food Sci.* **2016**, *8*, 33–42. [CrossRef]
50. Khang, D.T.; Dung, T.N.; Elzaawely, A.A.; Xuan, T.D. Phenolic profiles and antioxidant activity of germinated legumes. *Foods* **2016**, *5*, 27. [CrossRef] [PubMed]
51. Lee, M.; Hong, G.-E.; Zhang, H.; Yang, C.-Y.; Han, K.-H.; Mandal, P.K.; Lee, C.-H. Production of the isoflavone aglycone and antioxidant activities in black soymilk using fermentation with *Streptococcus thermophilus* S10. *Food Sci. Biotechnol.* **2015**, *24*, 537–544. [CrossRef]
52. Gosslau, A.; Li, S.; Ho, C.T.; Chen, K.Y.; Rawson, N.E. The importance of natural product characterization in studies of their anti-inflammatory activity. *Mol. Nutr. Food Res.* **2011**, *55*, 74–82. [CrossRef] [PubMed]
53. Amarowicz, R.; Shahidi, F. Antioxidant activity of faba bean extract and fractions thereof. *J. Food Bioact.* **2018**, *2*, 112–118.
54. Larkin, T.; Price, W.E.; Astheimer, L. The key importance of soy isoflavone bioavailability to understanding health benefits. *Crit. Rev. Food Sci. Nutr.* **2008**, *48*, 538–552. [CrossRef] [PubMed]
55. Rowland, I.; Faughnan, M.; Hoey, L.; Wähälä, K.; Williamson, G.; Cassidy, A. Bioavailability of phyto-oestrogens. *Br. J. Nutr.* **2003**, *89*, S45–S58. [CrossRef] [PubMed]

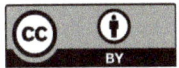

© 2018 by the authors. Licensee MDPI, Basel, Switzerland. This article is an open access article distributed under the terms and conditions of the Creative Commons Attribution (CC BY) license (http://creativecommons.org/licenses/by/4.0/).

MDPI
St. Alban-Anlage 66
4052 Basel
Switzerland
Tel. +41 61 683 77 34
Fax +41 61 302 89 18
www.mdpi.com

Foods Editorial Office
E-mail: foods@mdpi.com
www.mdpi.com/journal/foods

www.ingramcontent.com/pod-product-compliance
Lightning Source LLC
LaVergne TN
LVHW070541100526
838202LV00012B/347